When Matron Ruled

WHEN MATRON RULED

Peter Ardern

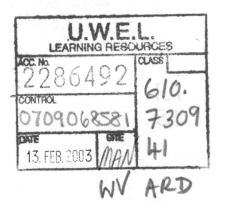

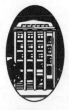

ROBERT HALE · LONDON

© *Peter Ardern 2002*
First published in Great Britain 2002

ISBN 0 7090 6858 1

Robert Hale Limited
Clerkenwell House
Clerkenwell Green
London EC1R 0HT

A catalogue record for this book is available from the British Library

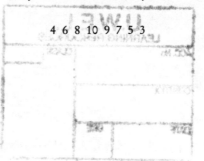

Typeset in 11/13 Garamond by
Derek Doyle & Associates, Liverpool.
Printed in Great Britain by
St Edmundsbury Press Limited, Bury St Edmunds
and bound by
Woolnough Bookbinding Limited, Irthlingborough

Contents

Acknowledgements

I wish to extend my thanks to all those who so generously gave their time to help in the writing of this book. In particular I would like to express my gratitude for the immense hospitality I received during the many visits I made for material. It was a privilege to meet with so many people who were prepared to share a life's experience with a virtual stranger.

Special thanks go to Julia Massey for her research support at the Institute of Naval Medicine, Gosport, and to Edith Curson and Gillian Comrey for their patient rewriting of material. I wish to thank also the staff of the Walsall Museum, Alex Attwell at the Florence Nightingale Museum (who is still keen to receive any new Nightingale material), and the staff of The Public Record Office, London, for their invaluable help. Thanks go also to the many hospitals and archive departments who provided information about matrons and staff both past and present. I would like to acknowledge my gratitude to the Emily MacManus family, in particular to her niece Maeve MacManus and great-nephew James MacManus. A special mention must go to Mike Owen for his enthusiastic support, and for putting me in touch with so many useful contacts. I would like to express my thanks to Lawrence Dopson (retired nursing journalist), and Pat Gould (retired QARNNS). I also owe a special debt to Lionel Lewis, Roy Stallard and Muriel Handley, Maria Brennan, Mrs Butterfield, Barbara Melrose, Mary Verrier, Norma Moore, and Betty Connor. Thanks are also extended to Linda Boland of Queensland, Australia, and Gloria Churchill of Boston, USA.

Thanks also to those who expressly wished to remain anonymous. Appreciation also to Richard Fuller, and to Barbara Samuels for her proofreading of the manuscript.

A special thank you must go to Sharon Thorpe for her invaluable advice and support throughout the writing of this book.

With the predominance of female interviewees of a high average age, it became quite clear that a chaperone would be of value. My wife June duly became involved, not only in this capacity, but also as a note-taker, secretary and supporter. I am indebted to her.

Finally, John Greene died during the writing of this book. It was a great pleasure to meet and talk with him, and I would like to extend my appreciation to his wife Betty and their two sons, Patrick and Kevin, for continuing to provide me with material from John's life and nursing career.

Foreword

Peter Ardern is to be congratulated on the timeliness of this excellent book given the current government imperative on 'Implementing the NHS Plan – Modern Matrons'. These guidelines recognize that positive role models and effective nursing leadership inevitably lead to better patient care. Implicit in this latest document is the value that is being placed by the government on the contribution of experienced nurses to healthcare.

Peter Ardern's book provides an important backdrop to these recent developments. It also enables us to appreciate the significant legacy entrusted to us by earlier leaders, which has formed the bedrock of nursing's past. Capturing the essence of this bedrock is essential to our understanding as we endeavour to shape our future with insight and sensitivity.

This insightful book will ensure that we do not lose sight of the centuries of experience that lie behind the role of contemporary nursing leaders. Whilst we may not always agree with the chain of events that our historical figures triggered, we should remember that they were of their time. These people put their heads above the healthcare parapet. They stood up to be counted . . . the buck inevitably stopped with them. They had the courage and they rightly deserve our respect and remembrance. Peter's interesting and informative work as enabled us to appreciate their legacy fully.

Having paid our dues in this celebration of nursing's past, we should now be in a better position to step forward with confidence and embrace new opportunities in the true spirit of turning political talk into professional action.

Roswyn A. Hakesley-Brown.
President of the Royal College of Nursing

Preface

The role of matron as nurse leader did not happen overnight; the job evolved over many centuries, with both the post and the post-holder influenced by a mixture of social attitudes, religion and military conflicts.

Anyone remembering Matron will have his or her unique memory of her. There are many descriptions of these remarkable nurse leaders. In her office she could be 'like a lion in its den, proud and imperious'; on her ward rounds she would be seen 'sweeping down the corridor and into the ward, for all the world like a diva about to assail the back of the auditorium with a grand Wagnerian aria'. These descriptions are very fanciful, but they tell us little about what the matron actually did and, just as importantly, who she was. In nursing history, the notion of 'matron' is already becoming remote from the younger generation. One of the matrons in this book explains that she was recently admitted to hospital, with her admission details being taken down by a young clerk. Asked about her previous work history, she replied that she had been a matron. The young lady looked very puzzled and enquired, 'What was a matron?'

In the nursing profession matron was the nurse leader. Easily identified by patients, visitors and staff alike, matron was also a professional, respected and experienced clinician, with the care of her patients at the centre of the profession she took pride in.

Often stereotyped as battleaxes or dragons, matrons already suffer from misrepresentation. If a history is not chronicled accurately, these myths will outlive reality. However the past is always with us; it is still embedded in the bricks and mortar of our hospitals. It is embedded in professional discipline and working practice, and we must remain conscious of this as we mould the future. With this in mind, it is my intention that this book should bring to the fore the wide range of matron's roles from the lesser-known to the famous.

Illustrations

Between pages 96 and 97

Between pages 192 and 193

21 Dr Robert and Mrs Mary Rose Wrangham on their wedding day, 1978
22 Lucy Baird on her twenty-first birthday in 1931
23 Miss J. Gillanders, matron 1946–59 with Miss Peterkins, sister tutor
24 Emily Soper, in her army sister uniform
25 Hilda Deacon, assistant matron, in 1939
26 Janet Baseley in bed in the children's ward, Royal Hospital, Portsmouth, Christmas 1960
27 Margaret Morris, Joan Churchhouse and Iris Cornforth, nurses at Miller Hospital, Greenwich
28 Lord Mayor Wyn Sutcliffe and Deputy Lady Mayoress Phyllis Lowe 1980–1
29 Staff of The Royal Hospital, Wolverhampton, in 1934
30 Miss Barbara Scott, matron, with HRH The Queen Mother at Queen Elizabeth Hospital, Birmingham, 1961
31 Kathleen Cooper, matron, with Peggy Nuttall, editor of *Nursing Times*, 1969
32 Maureen Fraser-Gamble, matron of Hammersmith Hospital, London, 1980
33 Marion Beveridge, matron of Hope Hospital, Salford, 1969
34 Miss Margaret Schurr, matron of Fulham Hospital, 1959
35 Ann Hirons, matron of Birmingham General Hospital receiving her MBE in 1987 accompanied by her brother, Dick, and sister-in-law, Ann
36 Miss Joyner, *c.* 1920, matron of a workhouse infirmary in Portsmouth

Credits

Walsall Local History Centre: 1. *Navy and Army Illustrated*: 2, 3. Author: 4. The Royal London Hospital Archives: 5, 6. Florence Nightingale Museum Archives: 7. Guy's Hospital: 8. Crown Copyright/MOD (Reproduced with the permission of the Controller of HMSO): 9, 10, 14, 15. Mary Butland: 11. David Lewis: 12. Betty Greene: 13. Commander Gillian Comrie: 16. Lionel Lewis: 17. Betty Connor: 18. Monica Matterson: 19. *Peterborough Citizen*: 20. Mary Rose Wrangham: 21. Lucy Baird: 22. Chris Farmer: 23. Emily Soper: 24. Betty Deacon: 25. Janet Gilbert: 26. Margaret Morris: 27. *The News*, Portsmouth: 28. Roy Stallard: 29. Barbara Scott: 30. Kathleen Cooper: 31. Maureen Fraser-Gamble: 32. Marion Beveridge: 33. Margaret Schurr: 34. Ann Hirons: 35. Mary Verrier: 36.

I
Woman's Work

Writing a book about nursing matrons means writing a history about women only, just as writing a book about physicians would mean writing a history involving men only. Well into the twentieth century heads of nursing were all female, answerable to heads of medicine still always male.

Man's first nurse was his mother. It was she who gave him security, food and warmth, who healed and nursed both child and man. Nursing and healing were synonymous. Throughout history women have acted as healers. They were 'silent' healers, because the woman as healer is an unwritten history, remaining unwritten because artefacts are not there offering evidence. History has been, in essence, a physical science where the study of remains and not people has predominated. Women's contribution to healing is more significant than historians have acknowledged. This is not surprising since, prior to the twentieth century, men wrote all histories and sciences, thus providing only male interpretations and descriptions.

For centuries, women have had to battle with social intolerance, educational restrictions, religious bigotry, witch hunts, and the prejudice and dogma of the medical profession. Any history of nursing has to be viewed against this background. That healing and nursing have their roots in ancient history there is no doubt, but what is questionable are the traditional roles males and females have played within this setting.

Primitive woman undoubtedly played a vital role in ensuring the welfare of herself, her husband and her children. Although hunting by the male provided an important source of food, the joint gathering of food provided a more reliable and safer way of sustaining the family's needs. Women were involved in the construction of shelters, the weaving of grasses, and tool-making, as well as food-gathering, cooking, child-care and garment-making. They were also involved in the medicinal application of plants and herbs.

As tribal life developed, people began to form into small, well-defined social units built around the nucleus of the family. In these early cultures it was normal for the mother to be the head of the family. Gradually her skills increased. Where she had been accustomed to using water for bathing and soothing, she began to use it as a healing medium. She recognized fire and heat as giving comfort; later she used it to cauterize wounds. Mixtures of herbs and other concoctions would have been the tools of these primitive healers.

Society became more settled and food supplies increased, allowing for the novel concept of 'leisure'. The man, relieved of the burden of merely surviving, began to travel, bringing back new knowledge. The woman could not compete in this; she did not have the freedom. Knowledge as a form of power was one of the early instruments of female repression; it was then that the husband and wife became unequal. This greater awareness of the world generated in men ideas that both terrified and excited them. Tribal leaders began to blame strange spirits for the devastating illnesses they were afflicted by. These illnesses were mysteries that went beyond man's understanding, so there was an increasing need for him to control them. The 'medicine man' or 'witch doctor' evolved to meet the challenge. When supernatural 'demons' were found to be the cause of ill health, they had to be exorcized in one of a variety of ways. Medicine was not a sophisticated art therefore it was seen to be of little use against 'unnatural' bodily invasions.

By the early and Middle Ages witch doctors had been replaced by religious leaders who still dabbled in mysticism, but the woman continued to heal; it was she who remained constant in developing the techniques of healing. As a healer she became more skilled in the use of herbal remedies, unguents and salves, passing formulae down from mother to daughter, and from female neighbour to female neighbour. Licensed doctors were available, but not in rural communities and small towns. The women of these villages and towns remained important both as healers and in fulfilling the roles of midwife and abortionist. Men were banned during childbirth; the presence of the husband, let alone another man, was considered inappropriate, distasteful or unlucky. Such a woman brought individuals into the world and witnessed them leave. She was indeed a 'wise woman'.

Women did not prosper well in other ancient civilisations, such as those in Egypt, India, Babylon and Palestine. Again they were held in rigidly defined social roles, which excluded them from working in the medical profession. Medicine was an exclusively religious domain, a pursuit of male priests. A woman's work was mainly confined to home-keeping and family business.

In Egyptian history during the pyramid age 2500–2000 BC, the first records appeared of men bearing the title 'physician' as distinct from that of 'magician'. Writings about physicians highlighted the 'maleness' of the role, but nursing *per se* received no mention. Indeed there is no mention of female nurses at all until the nineteenth century.

Women generally fared better in Rome. The influence of Christianity combined with Roman culture produced an environment in which women were held in higher esteem. Three women attained renown, namely Marcella, who turned her home into a monastery; Fabiola, who built a hospice and monastery, and Paula who also built a hospice for the sick. They remain the early matrons most often referred to. For each woman, a devotion to Christian beliefs allowed her access to the field of healing.

The first female healer to be written about was a Chinese woman named Ch'un Yu'yen. She was both midwife and provider of medicines for the queen of the Hans dynasty (260 BC–AD 220).

Back in Europe, men were becoming more prominent in medicine. A physical treatment, however, could not be conducted unless it was done in the presence of a religious man. Following the physical cure, the body of the patient would then be purged in order to remove evil spirits. Superstition and folklore continued to influence other strange 'cures', with professional physicians persisting in their bizarre beliefs and treatments even as late as during the nineteenth century.

Religion and nursing had become closely linked from the fifth century onwards. Monks and nuns were the only ones recognized as practising medicine and nursing; there was no organized medicine outside of the religious establishments. Hilda of Whitby founded a monastery in Yorkshire where she taught a mixture of medicine and nursing. In this monastic period, the division between medicine (male) and nursing (female) was not nearly so important because the priority of life in a monastery was prayer, not healing. Outside of the Church, women continued to pass on their knowledge of cures for physical ailments, their later male medical superiors adopting many of these.

The supply of medical treatments in medieval times could be subject to the prejudices of a class-ridden and divisive society. Great physicians did exist, but only to service the needs of the wealthy. The common man still required the services of the traditional female healer. Some of these women should have been considered great healers, but instead they received little, if any, recognition for their skills and were often described pejoratively as 'old wives'.

Most physicians were untrained and drug treatments were implemented without sound evidence that they were effective. Not until 1812 did the Royal College of Physicians begin to demand training for physicians, requiring them to have six months of hospital experience. From then on, the role of the male physician as an 'expert' was developed through the universities. The position gained extremely high status and was rigorously defended from intruders. For the new physicians, any other forms of treatment threatened their position of total authority. Their argument was that 'cures' from untrained females were 'dangerous nonsense', and from their lofty position of power, they reduced the role of the female healer to being regarded as little more than quackery, depicting them as amateur and unorthodox providers of folk medicine and nothing more. In this way women were excluded from practising their healing arts on the grounds of theology and education. At that time, Latin was the language of the universities where medicine was taught, and only men were permitted to receive this education.

Women healers came under even closer scrutiny from the fourteenth century until the seventeenth century not because of their skills but due to their confrontation with the Church. This was the time of the great witch-hunts. In Europe, the Bible injunction 'Thou shalt not suffer a witch to live' seemed to sanction widespread persecution. Women were accused of keeping and consorting with evil spirits, and other unholy pursuits. In England it was a difficult time for society and religion; for women healers in particular, it was a nightmare. The Malleus Maleficarum, written in 1485 by two German inquisitors, stated that apart from the crime of being female, a witch's other crime was that of healing. Medicine was, in reality, an emerging indistinct art, practised by a variety of men; physicians, barber-surgeons, apothecaries, alchemists, and untrained community healers all became authorities on medicine. For any woman practising these arts there were significant dangers, and a terrifying death at the stake awaited those accused of witchcraft.

By the end of the seventeenth century, only men could heal; it was on pain of death that women performed cures. This left a huge problem for the sick of the poorer classes who had relied on their wise women for treatments. The Church's answer to this was to endorse the notion that pain must be endured in deference to the suffering of Jesus, and that the patient's suffering would end through the release of death. The church was certainly not against medical care for the upper end of the social spectrum, however. The real issue was one of control: healing of the upper classes under the auspices of the Church and Crown was acceptable, whereas female healers working as part of a peasant subculture were not.

The Church's attack on peasant healers was essentially an attack on 'magical' healing. In a religious doctrine based on fear, the Devil was seen to have great power. According to the Church, women healers needed to evoke this power in order to be able to heal. Thus 'female' cures, even when successful, were not considered to be the work of God and even less the work of the healer because they were achieved through the help of the Devil. In this way, the act itself of curing was regarded as being evil.

Women healers had built up their healing powers through centuries of watching, listening, practising and learning from others. This only served to add weight to 'evidence' in support of witchcraft allegations. The woman's accusers were often those very physicians who sought to protect their own status. The mixing of potions was an obvious part of producing healing solutions and it is easy to see how this could be misinterpreted as more sinister actions. At witch trials, the physician was the expert, asked to decide on whether a 'cure' had been arrived at through magic, or knowledge of medicine. His judgement often became the deciding factor. As women were not deemed to have any knowledge of medicine, courtroom decisions inevitably went against them. 'If a woman dares to cure without having studied, she is a witch and must die.' It was to be many years before women recovered sufficiently to be able to establish themselves as professionals in nursing and, later, in medicine.

Many people believe that nursing really came into being following Florence Nightingale's work in the Crimea. Nothing could be further from the truth. The period between medieval times and the modern age was marked by two dramatic and powerful social trends: first of all, a decline in the influence of the Church, and secondly, an increasing belief in the immutable authority of science. Man no longer accepted a geocentric view of the universe, and scientific principles, once regarded as heresy, now challenged religious dogma.

As scientific law became established, magic and sorcery gave way to the new 'magic' of science. Gradually, the mysteries practised within medicine as it was then became redundant and observations were now made from a scientific viewpoint. The 1700s saw changes in how educated men saw the world. Now their experience went beyond superstition and myth to encompass the modern demands of scientific evidence. Whereas at the beginning of the seventeenth century a doctor's evidence could be used to establish guilt in witchcraft trials, by the end of that century this kind of testimony would have been unheard of. Although changes in society heralded a safer world for many would-be women healers, society most certainly did not provide women with better opportunities in the world of medicine.

By the twelfth century, three famous English hospitals had been established: St Bartholomew's, Bethlehem and St Thomas's. Each hospital has its particular place in history. The Bethlehem became noted for its care of the mentally ill and St Thomas's as the training school for Nightingale nurses. St Bartholomew's is of particular interest as it was the only one to remain open throughout nine centuries. During the Reformation, almost all of the hospitals in England were closed.

Rahere founded St Bartholomew's Hospital in London in 1123. He knew nothing about medicine or nursing care. With no knowledge of pathology or treatment, and no understanding of infection, a patient's recovery was doubtful. Medieval hospitals were religious establishments whose principal aim was to provide a comfortable environment for the sick in the hope that rest, regular meals and constant prayer would supply them with a cure. These institutions were small and could only accommodate a tiny proportion of those who needed care.

Throughout the monastic period members of the Augustinian order acted as nurses. They entered the order for the contemplation of a religious life, to serve God and to care for the sick. The person charged with the overall responsibility for the hospital was known as the 'Master', with nursing staff being referred to as 'Brothers' and 'Sisters'. An edict from the Bishop of London stated that the brothers and sisters should be 'diligent and pious in serving the sick'. They should also obey the master in carrying out care for the infirm, ensuring that no one was sent away unless they had recovered sufficiently.

The Reformation, or Protestant revolt, began on 31 October 1517 when Martin Luther nailed his ninety-five theses to the door of the Castle Church in Wittenburg. The theses attacked what he saw as the sale of papal indulgences. In 1536, despite Luther's excommunication and newly acquired outlaw status, his theological stance resulted in the dissolution of monasteries. The Reformation swept away monastic life in an attempt to reform the Roman Catholic Church. Unfortunately, and despite long records of charitable, medical and educational work, the hospitals also disappeared. Once again healing had to take place primarily in the patient's own home. In this way, the poor amongst the sick suffered even more during this period; there was no other provision for them. It was to be the eighteenth century before the growth of Voluntary Hospitals and Dispensaries emerged to serve their needs.

Thus began what is often referred to as a 'Dark Age' for nursing, and women's education in general. It is no coincidence that nursing and work for women began to be inextricably linked from this point on. Whilst medical science was advancing rapidly, the years up to 1860 saw conditions for England's nurses at their worst. The Reformation had already destroyed, to all intents and purposes, the only system of organized education for girls and young women. Women were once again excluded, restricted to servitude, and considered invalid as intellectual beings.

Conditions for the sick deteriorated so badly that King Henry VIII was compelled to refound St Thomas's Hospital, which was at that time attached to a priory. The master and the brothers were replaced by a President, Treasurer, and Board of Governors chosen from dignitaries of the City. In the late 1540s, a Royal Charter provided a new constitution for the hospital. The original forty-five beds were to be increased to one hundred, and medical staff were to be appointed with a matron and twelve women to make the beds, wash, and generally attend the sick. The very best of the hospitals and infirmaries of this time provided a relatively high quality of nursing; this is not always recognized by nurse historians. Due to ignorance of disease and infection, the work of matrons and the nurses was undertaken under the most difficult conditions.

The first known matron at St Bartholomew's Hospital was Rose Fisher. She was not the first matron in London however, the Savoy Hospital having a record of a matron appointed as early as 1526. Matrons of this period were generally held in high esteem and because they were considered to be of impeccable morals already, there was no official code of conduct. They were precisely what society expected of its 'ladies', and unlike ward sisters of the time, they were not subject to the rules of chastity and could be married. The matron's duties included receiving patients upon admission and placing them on the wards; she supervised the assistants and took responsibility for all the bedding; sisters and assistants were responsible to her, and no formal training was undertaken or required.

Not until the middle of the sixteenth did the first indication emerge of a specific role for the ward sister. This role simply entailed supplying practical daily living needs for patients. A few years later instructions for the ward sister's conduct were produced, stating that she should be gentle and diligent, obedient to matron, and faithful and charitable to the poor. More specifically their duties were to keep the patients clean, give them their food, make their beds, wash their clothes, and 'use unto them good and honest talk, such as may comfort them and amend them'. They were to avoid 'light, wanton and foolish words', scolding and drunkenness, and male company. Matron's permission was required if they were to leave their quarters, even to attend to a patient.

Sisters were expected to undertake all day-to-day 'domestic' work. Floors were strewn with rushes and patients lay on straw mattresses, which were burned when they became soiled. All transport to the wards of coal, food and drink was the duty of the ward sister. She emptied the slops, did the cleaning, and even whitewashed the walls. She also washed all the patients' clothing and bed linen. At St Bartholomew's Hospital, laundry was cleaned by pounding it in a large wooden vat known as the 'Buck'. This task, performed at three-weekly intervals, was called 'beating' the Buck. This duty came to be used as a selection criterion for promotion within the nursing ranks. Only those who had previously worked as nurses and performed duties 'at the Buck' could be eligible for appointment to Sister status.

By the 1670s, the first hierarchical structure was in operation in the leading hospitals. It was simple: Matron, Sister, Nurse and Helper. It was not until 1775 that Matron's duties and responsibilities were more clearly defined. The matron would take charge of the household goods and furniture, and she had to ensure the cleanliness of the bedchambers, beds, clothes, linen and everything else within the hospital. She would visit the wards and offices daily to see that the nurses, servants and patients observed the rules and did their duties. She would also check that the diets for patients were correct. Nurses and servants were expected to obey the matron 'as their mistress' and to behave with tenderness towards the patients and with civility and respect to visitors.

Matrons were generally widows of officers, the clergy or tradesmen, with their suitability based on their practical experience in matters of household management and the organisation of servants. Observance of social class and status formed an important aspect of the nursing hierarchy. There was a great deal of social division between the matron and her staff. Whilst the hospitals required their matrons to be women of a higher social class, this could not be said for the other grades of staff. Sisters and nurses were employed almost entirely on account of their physical strength since they had to undertake the heavy work such as washing and cleaning. As Matron was drawn from a higher social class than the other grades of staff, she represented the 'lady of the house' with the staff being merely servants. A ward sister could never be appointed to the post of matron, as sisters and nurses were not employed for their intellectual capabilities. Both matron and sister were placed in a masculine culture that demanded the highest feminine standards from them, at a time when many nurse reformers generally viewed nursing as contemptible. They were the archetypal 'ladies', the fairer sex; delicate, gentle, loving and dutiful.

Unfortunately for the nurses, the increasing expectations for and monitoring of the nurse role by boards of governors, along with the additional pressure of contact with young men (wounded soldiers and sailors), created an almost inexhaustible potential for disapproval. Negligence, extortion, theft, drunkenness, disorderly behaviour and keeping the company of men gave rise to summary dismissal. Other 'inappropriate' forms of behaviour, for example eavesdropping outside the governors' rooms, were regarded as disciplinary offences. Reformers were looking with an uncompromising eye for negative aspects of institutional care in order to highlight abuse, poor conditions and immoral behaviour, and they found plenty. Drinking practices were widespread throughout society and nursing was no exception. Nurses were constantly warned that they were forbidden to obtain money from patients, induce them to go to public houses, or consort with them. This behaviour was difficult to police since nurses would sleep in or next to the male dormitories.

All ward sisters and nurses lived in, and were subject to the behavioural restrictions of that institution. This included the necessity of gaining permission from Matron to be allowed out at night. While matrons were provided with their own apartments, ward sisters slept in specific areas set aside for them. Living conditions were generally basic and somewhat reminiscent of a convent lifestyle.

In 1771, Matron Susannah Robinson at St Bartholomew's Hospital reported to the Governors that she supervised 'upwards of one hundred' staff, including ward sisters and nurses as well as helpers and watchers, adding that 'the happiness and quiet of the patients greatly depends upon the qualifications and disposition of the persons employed to attend them'. She spent much of her time 'enquiring after their characters, interposing in ... disputes and squabbles between the sisters, nurses, helpers and patients, and removing the sisters and nurses into different wards as their capacities best suit'. Other housekeeping tasks were monitoring linen and laundry, ordering supplies, and ensuring patients were properly clothed. For these duties she received a yearly salary of £40, with a gratuity of £20. Matrons appointed from this period onwards were middle-class and had been used to running large households of servants where they exercised moral supervision and discipline, as well as teaching general hygiene principles. It was this quality that was desired when any matron post was offered.

Thirty years later, Mary Foot was elected Matron of St Bartholomew's Hospital. Her duties were now wider, but did not include nurse training. She was to receive all female patients on admission, allocate them a place, and attend the discharge of patients. She was also required to make a daily inspection of the wards, the laundry and the kitchen, making certain that the ward sister and nurses performed their duties appropriately. If ward sisters and nurses were not otherwise occupied, Matron set them to work mending sheets and bedding for the hospital.

By the middle of the eighteenth century major cities throughout Britain were building hospitals. The Public Infirmary in Manchester, forerunner to Manchester Royal Infirmary, opened in 1752. This was a small house with twelve beds. The first matron was Ann Worrall who stayed in that post for seven years. Although she had responsibility for twelve beds, she had received no training, nor did she have a trained nurse. She was later provided with a servant. Except for some expenses she was not paid at all for five months. She was then paid £3 and given a further £2 as a gratuity.

Decades after the initial distinction was made between matron, ward sister and nurse, the role of the nurse became more clearly separated. The nurse's duties comprised of general domestic tasks, making beds, washing pans and plates, and cleaning floors, beds and furniture. Nurses also collected bread, milk, provisions and warm drinks. They examined patients on admission (primarily for vermin), helped the patients in and out of bed, and cleaned the bedding of the incontinent patients. Their role evolved further as demands increased, and they began to assist the medical staff by administering fomentations (to relieve pain and inflammation), enemas and emetics. They attended surgical operations, offering comfort and support to the patient in the absence of anaesthetics. At night, nurses were required to place a clean chamber-pot under each bed, to take orders from the sister as to the nourishment needed by the patient, and to visit 'every weak patient's bedside' at least once an hour. On night duty they could be dismissed for allowing the ward fires to burn out or if they fell asleep.

By the 1830s, a ward sister at St Bartholomew's Hospital had greater responsibility than ever before. She was expected to carry out directions from the medical officers regarding the patients' diet and welfare, passing on relevant instructions to the nurses. She also reported any changes in a patient's condition to the medical staff. The administration of medicine was strictly the ward sister's domain and only in her absence would a nurse be authorized to carry out this function.

Religion still played a significant part in hospital life, with the Bible being regarded as the most suitable type of material for women to read. Many hospitals continued to adhere rigidly to their separate religions and any new staff had to be of that same denomination. Despite this emphasis on religion, many nurses in the nineteenth century were still viewed as ignorant, drunken and slovenly. Although this generalization was often true, in many cases it did a great injustice to those who provided good care in bad conditions.

To be sick and poor was undoubtedly a terrible situation, but this was nothing in comparison to life in the workhouse or workhouse infirmary. By the end of the nineteenth century most large cities had such infirmaries. They accommodated between five hundred and two thousand people at a time. The 'inmates' were destitute and homeless individuals of all ages.

Their meagre belongings were often stolen, along with their food, blankets and clothing. What little clothing they had was scarcely ever washed and insufferable misery largely went unrecognized. The workhouse infirmary model relied on female paupers nursing fellow mendicants, but this compulsory 'agreement' failed because most of the women were alcoholic prostitutes and unfamiliar with the notion of caring. Matrons of these establishments, wives of the masters recruited from the non-commissioned officer ranks in the military, frequently took the view that pauperism was a sickness in itself. The pauper nurse was distanced from the pauper in every way. She became a sort of moral guardian, transmitting the power to correct deviant behaviour, transforming the sickness and disharmony exhibited by paupers into an idealized image of social correctness, but she continued to be subordinate and obedient within the medical apparatus to sister, matron and the medical staff.

It was due to the pioneering work of people such as Miss Louisa Twining (1820-1912) that the visiting of workhouses began in 1853. Her persistence led to major changes in the workhouse system. These changes were taken up by the more enlightened masters and matrons, but it was to be the Nightingale matrons who, by introducing trained nurses, eventually replaced harsh practice with care and compassion.

In the census of 1851, the occupation of nursing was recorded as a form of domestic service. This labelling seriously maligned, but still reflected the contemporary opinion of, nursing work. However, by this time some outstanding women were doing heroic work nursing the sick. One such person was Sister Dora of Walsall.

Born Dorothy Wyndlow Pattison in Wensleydale on 16 January 1832, Dorothy had ambitions very early in life of nursing. Leaving school at the age of thirteen, she continued her intellectual development, encouraged by her family, and at thirty took up a teaching post. A new sisterhood was being formed at Coatham and, much to her father's disapproval, in 1864 she took the step of becoming Sister Dora. As Sister Dora, she began nursing at Middlesborough before being sent to Walsall. Here the severely sick and injured had to travel to Birmingham for hospital care and many died on the way. Throughout epidemics and disasters – it was an industrial area – Sister Dora was noted for playing a leading role in caring for the town's sick. One particular incident exemplifies the courage and dedication of this remarkable woman: twelve men were working in the furnace area at Birchills Foundry, Walsall, when there was a massive explosion. All the men were badly injured, suffering indescribable blast and burn injuries. Sister Dora forewent her bed for ten days to nurse these wounded men. Despite her best efforts, sadly only one man survived. In later years, she studied the antiseptic methods of Joseph Lister and learned more about surgical equipment prior to the opening of a new hospital in 1878.

There were many such women around the country who devoted their lives to nursing, but women remained systematically excluded from the high status of the medical profession in much the same way as they had been excluded from other learned professions. However, society was undergoing change, and women began to challenge the dominant role of men.

In 1849 Elizabeth Blackwell left England's shores and travelled to America to pursue her dream of a career in medicine. Although she had to overcome great difficulties in America, she had realized that her dream would have been unattainable in England. In the United States, she became the first woman to qualify as a medical doctor at the Geneva College in New York and graduated at the top of her class. However, her achievements came as a bitter blow to the masculine hierarchy of medicine. She had been admitted to the college as a joke, as a way of placating a feisty young woman, the men being secure in the knowledge that medicine would prove too difficult for her. Elizabeth's aptitude for her work provoked taunts and prejudice that plagued her throughout her time at the college. Shock and disbelief at her success generated resistance in academic circles, and it took Elizabeth's sister six years of persistence before she, too, was registered at the same college, albeit reluctantly.

In Edinburgh, the experiences of women attempting to breach the inner sanctum of medicine were awful. Fortunately these were women with indomitable spirit, who refused to be excluded. Among the medical students at Edinburgh was a formidable young woman called Sophia Jex-Blake. Born into a well-to-do and well-connected family in Hastings in 1840, she was determined to fight for the legal right of women to enter medical school as full-time students, and for them to take the qualifying examination of MD (Medical Doctor). In 1869 the Senate of Edinburgh University accepted Sophia, along with six other young women as full-time students. Now they were open to the most crass abuse both within the university itself and also in the streets. Male students chanted insults as they entered the gates and classes would be disrupted. Female intelligence once again proved too difficult for male colleagues to cope with when one of the women students had the 'audacity' to gain the highest marks for an examination. She should have been awarded the Hope Scholarship for Chemistry but instead the accolade went to the male candidate who came second. Accusations of discrimination were levelled at the University when this became known outside. The success of these young women only served to exacerbate problems for female students. Professors refused to lecture them and a riot by male students, fuelled by fear and anger, culminated in an attack of insults and obscenities directed towards women.

Following this experience it became obvious to Sophia Jex-Blake that even if women were allowed to continue training, they may not be allowed to gain their medical degree. Unable and unwilling to accept defeat, she took her case to the law in 1872 and won the right for women to take the MD degree examination. On 17 October 1887, Dr Sophia Jex-Blake opened the first hospital in Scotland to admit female medical students. This was Leith Hospital, which had originally been established in the fifteenth century. With the assistance of Elizabeth Garrett Anderson, a Bill was passed in 1876 permitting all degree-granted medical institutions and bodies to admit women to their examinations. A year later the Royal

Free Hospital in London also allowed women to receive practical training in its wards.

For other women the only way they could advance in medicine was through nursing. In this field it was possible to achieve more prestige and responsibility. The task now was twofold: getting the right person to be head of the nurse hierarchy, and attracting the right sort of people into nursing. Where were such people to be found? The matron needed to be trained and nurses could no longer be drawn from the servant classes. This problem was recognized by Florence Nightingale even before she returned from the Crimea. Nursing needed to be transformed into a new kind of occupation, to catch up with the developments in medicine and changes in society.

II

Angels of the Crimea

The Crimean War was fought from 1853 to 1856 between the Russians and the British, French and Ottoman alliance. It started as a squabble amongst politicians over Black Sea trade routes, but developed into war on a scale never seen before. Nearly 20,000 British soldiers were lost, not only killed directly by a combination of weaponry and strategies, but mainly through archaic and ignorant medical practices. Disease, neglect and appalling conditions within the hospitals claimed many of these men's lives.

Sergeant-Major Timothy Gowing was severely wounded in battle by a bayonet. He described the awful conditions on board a hospital ship transporting the wounded to hospital. He spoke of a ship rolling and tossing about at sea full of wounded soldiers. The sight was heart-breaking. The wounded had not received any medical care since their injuries and there was none available on board ship. They had fought for their country and were likely to die in agony, and worse was to come. Instead of being met on arrival by medical and nursing teams they were greeted by confusion and disorder. Arriving at Scutari Hospital there was still no relief, as it was overflowing with wounded men. They had to endure another sea journey to Malta, but at least in Malta he gave a glowing account of the care he received from the female nurses there.

For the first time, war became a highly public event. Widespread use of the telegraph and the arrival of the 'war correspondent' enabled a relatively uncensored account of the war to be broadcast. Detailed descriptions of the tremendous suffering caused public outrage, not least from Queen Victoria, who was said to be so moved by the suffering that she was instrumental in the hurried building of Netley Hospital for wounded soldiers. These reports also focused the attention of medical professionals, galvanizing them into action. Men and women worked side by side to try to reduce the appalling loss of life and, for the first time, the contribution of female nurses and their heroism, determination and courage were positively reported.

This brief and bloody time bore witness to the deeds of many remarkable people. Among them were Mrs Mackenzie, Elizabeth Davis, Mary Jane Seacole and, of course, Florence Nightingale. Into the hell that was the Crimea these women brought order, cleanliness, basic necessities and humanity. Florence Nightingale, already a highly respected character in nursing, was dispatched by the British government to inspect the conditions at Scutari Hospital and other hospitals in the Crimea. She took with her a party of thirty-eight women, consisting of twenty-four Sisters of religious orders and fourteen practical nurses. Nightingale had exacting standards, and for this reason it had been no easy task for her to muster this number of suitable staff. Among them were Sarah Ann Tarrot, Anne Ward Morton, and Mary Barker. It is said that authority and discipline were needed to deal with differences in social status, education and varying religious beliefs.

Following their arrival on 4 November 1854, the group led by Miss Nightingale set to work. The base hospital was over-crowded and filthy. Eighteen hundred casualties struggled for survival in cold draughty wards. Ventilation was grossly inadequate and vermin ran free. There was little comfort for the wounded and patients had to lie on the floor virtually where they fell, without sheets or blankets. There were few medical supplies, no clean water, no facilities for basic hygiene, inadequate sewage disposal, and notorious neglect of the areas for food preparation. Dysentery, fever and infection were rife. This was not a place for healing; it was a place to die.

Miss Nightingale swept into the fray, angry and poised for

attack. She immediately encountered open hostility and exclusion from many of the medical staff, and she became a constant irritation to the hospital hierarchy. It was due to her firm belief in her purpose and the enormous influx of casualties that made the medical staff finally accept her. She wrote many letters to England describing the medical and nursing conditions. Her intentions were to generate sympathy for her cause. With the journalistic support of W.H. Russell, a *Times* reporter, she utilized the power of negative publicity to get her message across, writing about the terrible circumstances of the wounded soldiers, their treatment and the mismanagement of resources. A leading article in *The Times* of 23 December 1854 identified the difficulties.

> Incompetence, lethargy, aristocratic *hauteur*, official indifference, favour, routine, perverseness and stupidity reign, revel and riot in the camp before Sebastopol, in the harbour of Balaclava, in the hospitals of Scutari, and how much nearer to home we do not venture to say.

Without question Miss Nightingale transformed conditions at Scutari. Her first task was to organize staff. There were only two or three nurses per hundred patients, so they could not possibly have managed without considerable help. A great deal of this help came from the male orderlies and soldiers' wives, but they were given little or no credit. As with other military establishments, the work was arduous and performed under extreme conditions.

At the hospital, Miss Nightingale and her staff had to tackle the immediate problems of reorganising space, increasing food rations and supplying new equipment, clothing and medical supplies. These were not easy tasks as at that time the army had a system of ordering that was very bureaucratic – she needed three signatures to order any item. This was not deliberate intransigence on the part of the army; they were just as badly served because non-military personnel controlled all ordnance. Nightingale also had to fight a difficult battle to improve ever aspect of the patients' lives. In doing so, the number of deaths was dramatically reduced. Miss Nightingale also concerned herself with the rehabilitation of patients, setting up reading rooms and a canteen, even writing letters home to their loved ones. These dramatic reforms came at a price however, especially for the nurses. One hundred and twenty five women worked for Florence Nightingale and it was an extremely hard life for them. Miss Nightingale was forceful, ruthless and demanding of both those in authority and those in obedience. She simply would not tolerate anything but perfection.

Nurse Sarah Ann Terrot was one of the Sellonite Sisters in Miss Nightingale's party at Scutari. Speaking glowingly at all times of Miss Nightingale, Sarah Ann kept a diary of her experiences of disease, exposure, malnutrition, terror and organizational chaos in the Crimea. She recorded in detail the horrendous conditions they had found on entering Scutari Hospital. She also noted things such as doctors having to sign requisition forms before being handed a towel. She was appalled that men were stripped of their shirts before being buried – having already undergone neglect, deprivation, fatigue, cold and hunger, this was the final insult. Her personal interest in the welfare of the soldiers is striking when one considers the harshness of the conditions she worked in. She received the Royal Red Cross from Queen Victoria in 1897.

Although not a nurse herself, Mrs Mackenzie was charged by the Royal Navy with managing the nursing staff at Therapia Hospital where injured sailors and marines were taken from the front line at Sebastopol. Mrs Mackenzie offered her services in November 1854 and quickly gathered a group of nurses to assist her. Although she had studied hospital management at the Middlesex Hospital, she felt she needed to prepare herself for the rigours of trauma nursing. As a measure of the bravery of this woman, and indeed many women of this time, she deliberately exposed herself to the rigours of attending a surgical operation at St Thomas's Hospital, London. Here, despite the availability of chloroform, she witnessed an above knee amputation done without anaesthetic. The anger she felt from this brief experience was to stay with her forever. She believed that her rage had prevented her from being sick and fainting.

Following this ordeal, and with understandable hesitation, Mrs Mackenzie accepted the posting to Therapia, writing:

> It is now settled that we go to Therapia taking six nurses, and that I have the charge and management of the female department there. Also, the Admiralty wish to make female nursing general throughout their hospitals if it is successful at Therapia. This responsibility is truly awful, but I have been inclined to undertake it because it appears to be most difficult to get anybody who will go out without settling so much about creeds and confession – nay, about gowns and bonnets – while sailors and Marines are now lying in a deplorable state. My only dread is the increased responsibility, for I am to be the Miss Nightingale of Therapia.[1]

Mrs Mackenzie arrived at Therapia with her husband Revd John Mackenzie and a party of nurses in January 1855. All her nurses proved to be quite remarkable. They included Miss Erskine and Miss Veysie, who had both been rejected as unsuitable for Miss Nightingale's party. All of the nurses were praised by Dr Davidson, the Deputy-Inspector in charge of the hospital, both for their kindness to the patients and for their refusal to shrink from any kind of duty. Being members of the 'fairer sex', they were not expected to withstand the arduous conditions, but this group of nurses surprised even the harshest and most sceptical critics. The hospital at Therapia treated cholera, scurvy and frostbite, as well as wounds from conflict. In the Crimea, whereas one soldier would die from his wounds, another nine would die of disease.

Having a smaller staff and hospital than Miss Nightingale, Mrs Mackenzie did not have to deal with as many problems. She was accepted almost immediately by the medical staff and enjoyed glowing tributes for the work she and her nurses undertook, and was made an honorary member of the officers' mess. The Inspector of Hospitals wrote that: 'Mrs Mackenzie's management continues to be admirable, and the devotion of her nurses untiring, while, with one exception only, the conduct of the paid female nurses is most praiseworthy.' She was undoubtedly fortunate with her nurses, none having to return to England on account of misdemeanours. Although there were problems with requisitioning stores, Mrs Mackenzie overcame this with patience and tact. During an inspection of Therapia Hospital, Miss Nightingale herself fell ill and was nursed by Mrs Mackenzie.

After two years of devotion to the staff and patients of Therapia, Mrs Mackenzie's health declined and she was forced to return to England in November 1857, where retirement from nursing awaited her. She left her hospital in the capable hands of Miss Erskine and Miss Veysie who remained, continuing the work, until the termination of hostilities. Their work would long stay in the grateful remembrance of the officers, seamen and marines who fought at Sebastopol. As a lasting tribute to Mrs Mackenzie, and her contribution in laying the foundations at Therapia for the future establishment of QARNNS, the Nurses' Mess at Haslar Hospital, Gosport, is named after her.

Elizabeth Davis was a well-travelled and fiercely independent Welsh woman who was already in her sixtieth year when she went to Scutari. She was renowned for both her nursing and her cooking skills. Her kitchen at the Crimea was long remembered by soldiers. She quickly found harrowing examples of neglect. One soldier had been wounded at Alma by a shot that had caused extensive chest and arm injuries. The wound had not been dressed for five weeks and Miss Davis 'took at least a quart of maggots from it'. She removed them by the handful from many of the other wounded as well. Once the wounds were regularly attended to, these men soon got well. Having done a considerable amount of nursing she knew that there should be no such infestation in wounds that are properly cleaned and dressed. She rightly considered their presence a proof of neglect.

Miss Davis and Miss Nightingale had a notoriously difficult relationship, full of disagreement and hostility. A rigid sense of justice and fair play led Miss Davis to criticize the behaviour of her superior. She alleged that at Scutari, Miss Nightingale had preferential treatment with a French cook employed to prepare her food. She was also appalled by Miss Nightingale's strict adherence to the complex army system of requisitioning food and clothing. The following highlights the tone of that relationship:

> It occurred when Miss Davis wanted to move on from Scutari hospital to the Crimea to be nearer the fighting. She felt she could do more good for the wounded if they were treated before the long journey to Scutari! Unfortunately Miss Nightingale did not agree. The two had a notoriously difficult relationship. Miss Davis did not like being at Scutari and Miss Nightingale would not brook dissent. She sent for Miss Davis and explained her objections, but these were not accepted. Miss Davis stuck to her guns that her rightful place was at the front. She allowed her to go with the parting shot that if she misbehaved at the Crimea there would be no home for her at Scutari and that she would be sent back to England. This got Miss Davis's blood up, replying that neither man nor woman dared to accuse her of misbehaving. Miss Davis was a success at the Crimea particularly because her kitchen was second to none. Sadly, she ended her life destitute after having been a significant figure both at the Crimea and in other serving roles around the world. Like many women she was not rewarded for the efforts she had made. She died in 1860 at the age of seventy-one.

Mary Jane Seacole was a West Indian nurse and 'doctress'. She learned the art of healing from her mother who ran a boarding house for invalid soldiers. Mary earned the respect of the British regiments and was affectionately known as 'Mother'. When she discovered what was happening in the Crimea, she tried to join the Nightingale nurses, but was rejected. It was likely that her nationality had some part in the decision. Despite this rebuke, her healing instincts compelled her to go to the Crimea, even though she had to pay for her own passage.

Her initial reaction to Scutari was shock – she could hardly believe the amount of suffering that faced her. Miles of corridors throughout the hospital were littered with injured men, dying and some already dead, but like Miss Davis she realized that if it was like this at Scutari, it must have been so much worse at the front. With this in mind she decided that the place for her was at the front, where the suffering was bound to be greater. On the very first day that she approached the wharf, a party of sick and wounded had just arrived. With so many patients, she felt sure that the doctors would be glad of all the help they could get. So strong was her impulse to help that she did not wait for permission and immediately set to work. As she already had nursing skills, she was able to help immediately.

W.H. Russell wrote about her unfailing bravery and skill. He had seen Mrs Seacole set off under fire with her little store of creature comforts for the wounded men, 'and a more tender and skilful hand about a wound or broken limb could not be found among our best surgeons'. Mrs Seacole was also noted for her hospitality and she supported the soldiers by providing extra provisions for them. Russell also noted that he had seen her at the fall of Sebastopol laden not with plunder, the 'good old soul', but with wine, bandages and food for the wounded and the prisoners.

In recognition of her work at the Crimea, and the fact that she was made bankrupt due to the changing fortunes of war, *Punch* magazine raised funds so that she would not suffer financially from her efforts.

What the medical profession had regarded as the inevitability of war, these nursing women saw as an abomination. Working for the benefit of humankind, their good work shone brightly amidst the chaos of war, but for the most part, sadly, their invaluable contributions slipped into historic oblivion.

Without a doubt, Florence Nightingale stole the limelight. She was viewed as a ministering angel, a woman of courage, and also a great reformer. Miss Nightingale had many advantages not least because she was a well-connected woman of independent means. She was a prolific letter-writer and a powerful campaigner, throughout her life. She is credited with single-handedly leading a campaign that revolutionized nursing. She never allowed herself to forget how she stood on the filthy floors, dressing maggot-infected wounds and attending amputations, listening to the screams of the victims, seeing men unable to cleaned or be given fresh linen for their wounds or bedding, watching men die. Nightingale vowed that she was never going to accept such conditions again. She changed nursing forever from a mucky and careless containment of injured people, to a managed care system based on solid principles of health promotion.

On her return to England, Florence Nightingale was still only thirty-six years old, but was soon to become acknowledged as the supreme authority on hospitals and their construction. A genius at administration and organization, she was to revolutionize the way hospitals were run. The sanitary measures she introduced at Scutari Hospital were exemplary, and she substituted administrative chaos with decency and order. No one can fully appreciate the effect this woman had on the health and welfare of ordinary people, but what was Nightingale like as a person and how did she come to play such an important role in the Crimea?

Born in Florence, Italy, on 12 May 1820, Florence Nightingale began her 'career' in Paris, studying the work of the Sisters of Charity, then spending three months at the Kaiserswerth Deaconesses Institute, Germany. At the Institute, Pastor Fliedner and his wife Friederike taught a three-year nursing course including both bedside and classroom instruction. These experiences were to have a profound effect on the futures of Miss Nightingale and of nursing. Her first opportunity to apply her knowledge was as a superintendent at an institution in Harley Street, London. This was a benevolent institution offering shelter and nursing care to homeless women and sick 'governesses'.

Nightingale had prepared herself since the age of seventeen for some sort of social care role, but parental resistance had prevented any such opportunities so far. She was, without doubt, a highly complex person; extremely hard-working to the point of being fanatical, she could be skittish one moment severe the next. Deeply religious, she invoked God in her correspondence sometimes inappropriately. She would address her probationers, whom she encouraged to write to her, as the 'Pearl' or 'Goddess-Baby'. She would also encourage probationers, sisters and matrons to write to her about their own colleagues and seniors, thus creating a unique network of information. It could be said that Nightingale was very attention-seeking, but she took to her bed for much of her later life, mostly shunning public accolade. Sir Sidney Herbert, then Secretary of State for War, was the main influence in setting her up for her major role in transforming nursing. It was Herbert who recognized the ability this woman had, not only in taking on the great task at Scutari but also in establishing nursing as a reputable occupation. Florence Nightingale died on 13 August 1910 and is commemorated annually at St Paul's Cathedral.

To understand fully the accomplishment of Miss Nightingale, it is also important to recognize the differences of the age in which she lived. When she returned to England the task ahead of her was to be as difficult as the Crimea. Many hospitals were still places of wretchedness, degradation and squalor. Hospital 'smell', the result of dirt and lack of sanitation, was accepted as unavoidable, and was so overpowering that people entering wards for the first time were seized with nausea. Wards were usually large, bare and gloomy; bed space was cramped with as many as fifty or sixty beds crowded into a single ward, each bed having less than two feet of space between it and the next one so there was no privacy for the patients, nor was there any for the nurses. It was not uncommon for nurses to sleep in the wards they nursed on, even in the male wards if that was where they were assigned.

At this time there was no treatment for cancer and it had to run its inevitable course; the pain and suffering had to be endured with only minimal relief. To nurse these people with their bodies rotting must have been almost unbearable.

Inadequate hospital facilities and the lack of properly trained staff meant that reliance on prayers was still necessary. In many of the large cities the patients came from slum tenements, hovels and cellars where cholera was a constant threat. It was common practice to put a new patient into the same bedlinen used by the last occupant, and as mattresses were generally made of flock, they were sodden and seldom, if ever, cleaned. These physically disgusting conditions were not the only obstacles in Nightingale's purpose to reform nursing – she highlighted the major problem as the lack of suitable nurses.

Nightingale's reforms began in 1860 with money raised to commemorate her work in the Crimea. Her first objective was to open a training school for nurses. Fortunately, after the experience of the Crimea, the medical establishment and the government had to recognize the significant role that nursing had played in reducing casualties. To spearhead her reforms Miss Nightingale needed help from a new, professional class of trained nurse leader – Matron.

Note

1 Mrs John Mackenzie, quoted in Penney, M.E. 'The Miss Nightingale of Therapia' (*Nursing Times*, 25 September 1954).

III
Nightingale's Matrons

Never a matron herself, Florence Nightingale was clear about the type of person she wanted to train as a nurse leader. The type of 'lady' Miss Nightingale envisaged was a middle-class woman used to looking after and managing a household of servants. Not yet emancipated in wider society, within their own homes these women had authority. They organized and ran the day-to-day functions of the home, and exercised moral supervision over the female staff. They also enforced discipline and respect, values essential for successful nursing. These potential nurse leaders were to go into large, male-dominated institutions to reorganize outdated systems, change antisocial practices, develop nursing policies and break down years of prejudice against women, illness and poverty. These women had to be from a class that was respected and was used to being respected. They were to be trained as nurses but act like managers. They were to be the pioneers of hospital reform. What set the Nightingale School above all other institutions was this idea of being trained for a job. At this time it was still not considered appropriate in nursing, teaching, or any other profession in which women worked.

The Nightingale School for Nurses was opened at St Thomas's Hospital in Southwark on 24 June 1860. An advertisement had been placed in *The Times* in May 1860 inviting applications. Applicants were divided into probationers and paying-probationers, the latter group expected to take higher posts at St Thomas's and other hospitals. Recruits were not easy to find and were chosen with great care. Accommodated in a special building which was situated in the centre of the 'Gardens' adjoining the hospital, they had separate bedrooms and a common sitting-room. Close by were two rooms allocated to the sister in charge. A basic principle underlying the development of the school was that there were to be two grades of pupils: educated probationers forming the upper class would pay about thirty pounds a year for tuition; a non-paying group, selected for 'fitness and character', would be representative of the less-educated. A non-paying probationer in her first year was paid usually at the rate of £1 a month. The pay of fully trained nurses in the hospital ranged from £20 to £40. Sisters usually received between £35 and £60. Board, lodging and sometimes articles of clothing were provided free. The salary of a matron was upwards of £300.

St. Thomas's Hospital was not then the well-lit and accessible place it is now. A visitor generally would have to get to it by a horse-drawn vehicle ridden through some of the more dimly lit riverside streets surrounding the hospital. The Thames flowed nearby, carrying with it much of London's refuse (well-described in Dickens's novel, *Our Mutual Friend*). It wasn't safe for a man – let alone a woman – to venture out alone at night. Agnes Jones, a future matron, was one of the first fee-paying Nightingale Probationers. She was thirty years of age when she began her training in 1862. It must have been an anxious time for any new Nightingale nurse as she travelled through London towards St Thomas's Hospital. Miss Jones, although a mature woman, would have known little about what she was to expect as a trainee nurse.

Turning along the river at Southwark, the trainee would face the huge gates of St Thomas's Hospital. Ringing the bell to announce herself, she would initially have been greeted by the porter. On entering the courtyard in a horse-drawn cab along with her luggage, she would be admitted into a large warm hall. The hall in those days was a grand room, wood-panelled and partitioned. The floor and walls were varnished, highly polished and very clean. She would wait there while the cab driver unloaded and brought in her luggage. The porter would then escort her to a small inner hall. Depending on the time of day, Mrs Wardroper would be there to meet her or otherwise there would be 'deaconess-looking' nurses to greet her. She would then be escorted through the hospital, catching glimpses of the wards and the open spaces filled with trees, to an area for refreshments before being escorted to the 'cell' where she was to reside throughout her training at the school. The cell would contain a bed, a small chest of drawers, wash-stand, chair and towel rail.

Like Miss Jones, the trainees were to be given board and their own lodgings and be supervised by a sister. They were to be given instruction in the wards by the Superintending Sisters, the Matron and Residential Medical Officer. The following are the conditions for admission and instruction for probationers:

1. The Committee for the Nightingale Fund have made arrangements with the Authorities of St Thomas's Hospital for giving a year's training to women who wish to be employed as hospital nurses.
2. Ladies wishing to undertake training of this nature should apply to the Matron of St Thomas's Hospital, Mrs Wardroper, who is authorized to decide whether they should be received as probationers at the Hospital. The age considered suitable for the trainees is between 25 and 35. Date of birth and good character should be certified on a form drawn up by Mrs Wardroper, and a doctor's certificate with his name and address is also required.
3. The probationers are to obey the Matron and to observe the rules of the Hospital.
4. They are to have their own lodgings in the Hospital, board (including tea and sugar) and washing, which is all to be paid for by the Fund, and they will be given a certain number of articles of clothing of a uniform cut which they will be obliged always to wear inside the Hospital. They are to serve as assistant nurses in the wards of the Hospital.
5. They are to be instructed by the nurses (Sisters) and the Superintendent. At the end of the first quarter they are to

be paid the sum of £2, at the end of the second quarter £2.10s, at the end of the third quarter the sum of £3.

6. After one year their period of training shall be considered complete and they will then be obliged to enter into service as hospital nurses and to accept such posts as may be offered them.

7. The names of the probationers are to be entered in a register in which notes are to be made concerning their conduct and their various degrees of skill. At the end of each month this register is to be shown to the trustees of the Nightingale Fund. After one year such probationers as have been found by the Committee to have acquitted themselves in a satisfactory manner as regards the instruction and the training, are to be entered into the register as qualified nurses and accordingly to be recommended for posts as such.

8. The period of training for a pupil shall be one year, and she is to be admitted on the clear understanding that she is expected to remain for the whole of this period. However, for reasons accepted by the Council, pupils may be allowed to leave the course at three months' notice. They may at any time be sent away by the Matron because of misconduct or if she should find them unsuitable or careless in the discharge of their duties. After examination they shall be considered qualified for regular posts as extra nurses at St Thomas's either in the course of the training year or at the end of it. The Council is confident that it will be able to provide posts for its certified nurses, either at St Thomas's or at some other hospital.

9. On the presentation of a certificate of their having served satisfactorily in a hospital for one entire year subsequent to that of their training, the Council offers gratuities of £5 and £3 (according to two classes of efficiency) to its certified nurses.

10. The first quarter of each training year begins on June 24. Applications should be made to the Matron of St. Thomas's Hospital, Newington, London South, between 10 and 11 a.m. if the applicant wishes to hand in her appli-

cation in person [note that there was no expectation of male applicants].

The training was almost exclusively practical and included everything that a nurse was expected to understand and be able to do at a sickbed. The duties of a probationer were quite straightforward:

The pupil must be sober, honest, trustworthy, punctual, quiet and orderly, cleanly and neat. It is her duty to acquire skill:

1. In the dressing of blisters, burns, sores, wounds, and in applying fomentations, poultices, and minor dressings.
2. In the application of leeches, externally and internally.
3. In the administration of enemas for men and women.
4. In the management of trusses, and appliances in uterine complaints.
5. In the best method of friction to the body and extremities.
6. In the management of helpless patients, i.e. moving, changing, personal cleanliness of, feeding, keeping warm (or cool), preventing and dressing bed sores, managing position of.
7. In bandaging, making bandaging and rollers, lining of splints, etc.
8. In making the beds of the patients, and removal of sheets whilst patient is in bed.
9. She is required to attend at operations.
10. To be competent to cook gruel, arrowroot, egg flip, puddings, drinks for the sick.
11. To understand ventilation, or keeping the ward fresh by night as well as by day; she must be careful that great cleanliness is observed in all the utensils, those used for secretions as well as those required for cooking.
12. To make strict observation of the sick in the following particulars: the state of secretion, expectoration, pulse, skin, appetite, intelligence, as delirium or stupor; breathing, sleep, state of wounds, eruption, formation of matter, effect of diet or of stimulants, and of medicines.
13. And to learn the management of convalescents.

Certainly there were teething troubles plaguing the early years of the Nightingale School. There was a general lack of commitment from the sisters who were supposed to supervise the pupils – this problem persisted despite attempts by both Miss Nightingale and Mrs Wardroper to resolve it – and the pupils' handwriting was not always as good as it should have been. There were also constant restrictions on what a nurse could or could not do.

Rebecca Strong, a future matron of the Royal Hospital Glasgow, who trained in 1867, recalled that it was the medical students who took temperatures and pulses and tested urine and that few records were kept. Personal cleanliness and kindness were stressed. These were times when, for example, a dislocation of the shoulder was remedied by ropes being attached at one end to two or three of the supporting pillars of the first floor, and the other end to the patient's shoulder. Each student was in charge of a rope and at a word of command, the students would give a jerk which apparently proved successful in most cases. Kindness was indeed a highly valued commodity!

Training for the probationers consisted initially of emphasizing the importance of one's character as much as technical training. Hence the school was said to have begun with an almost missionary ardour and selfless devotion the keys. The basic plan for the school was that the Nightingale Fund would pay for the matron, ward sisters and medical lectures. St. Thomas's Hospital was chosen because it had medical school connections, and a tradition of care for the sick dating back for centuries. Mrs Wardroper was previously known to Miss Nightingale through her involvement in providing nurses for the Crimea, and for this reason she was deemed most suitable for the position of Matron.

Of the 148 Nightingale nurses who entered training between 1860 and 1870, seventeen were dismissed for reasons ranging from ill health and disobedience, to insobriety and incompetence. By the end of 1870, twenty-six women had become 'Lady Superintendent' or 'Matron' in Britain or abroad.

Mrs Sarah Wardroper (1822-92) could be described as the first, or pioneer, matron of modern times. Many nursing historians describe her as a remarkable person to whom the success of the Nightingale School is almost entirely due. She was left a widow with four children. She gained the post of Matron of St Thomas's on 14 February 1854, remaining in the post for thirty-three years. Without doubt Miss Nightingale had the greatest respect for Mrs Wardroper. She was inclined to marvel at her achievements, at what she had done rather than at what she had not done. She saw her at that time as a hospital genius, managing St Thomas's better than anyone else could have done. It must be remembered as well that Mrs Wardroper was neither backed up by good quality trained staff, nor did she have an assistant.

Mrs Wardroper was the powerhouse behind both the reforms at St Thomas's and at the training school, and deserves considerable credit for this. She began the reforms in one part of the hospital and then extended them to other areas, a method that was subsequently incorporated by the graduates of the training school. Her greatest skill was at hospital organization. Miss Crossland, the home sister and tutor from 1873 to 1896, was also highly significant in the success of the training school; she was an outstanding teacher. Working closely with Mrs Wardroper, Miss Crossland taught a wide range of medical, nursing and even ethical and religious subjects, as well as literacy skills, which many pupils needed.

Mr R.G. Whitfield, the Resident Medical Officer, also had the greatest respect for Mrs Wardroper. In September 1868 he wrote about the great reforms and the new controlling power held by the matron over the sisters and nurses. Although this was greatly disliked by individual medical officers, it was proving a successful system. He found that Mrs Wardroper had 'outlived' all opposition, and pronounced that both publicly and privately she was a great success.

Sarah Wardroper was an educated women, unlike many of her predecessors. Her personal appearance was described as striking; she was tall and dark, and possessed a personal magnetism which enabled her to impart discipline. She had great powers of administration, was a tireless worker, and an ardent reformer. She was also a strict disciplinarian and excellent teacher. Miss Nightingale described her as 'straightforward and true, free from artificiality and self-interest ... She never went "a-pleasuring" and was seldom in society.' Although Mrs Wardroper was not a 'trained nurse' herself, the probationers who went through the school had the greatest respect for her. One such probationer, whose father was a high-ranking army officer, related this respect in the following way. Regarding her father's meeting with Mrs Wardroper, the pupil nurse 'could not have been more pleased than if he had been meeting with the queen'.

Every month Mrs Wardroper filled in personal reports about the pupils entitled 'Personal Character and Acquirement'; by this she exercised very close supervision over every probationer. The details of the report were minutely and comprehensively detailed with two main headings. 'Moral Record' and 'Technical Record'. The Moral Record had six subdivisions – punctuality, quietness, trustworthiness, personal neatness, cleanliness, and ward management and order. The Technical Record had fourteen subdivisions, which were themselves subdivided, in some cases having yet further subdivisions. She graded each probationer as 'excellent', 'good', 'moderate', 'imperfect', or '0' [zero]. Confidential reports were also kept and sent to Miss Nightingale. A daily diary was written by each student so that Miss Nightingale could follow the probationers' progress; from these she noted some very lax spelling and so arranged for extra spelling lessons.

Both Miss Nightingale and Mrs Wardroper had dominant personalities that occasionally clashed. After the inaugural period was over, their differences, as might have been foreseen, became more marked with Miss Nightingale constantly doubting Mrs Wardroper's abilities. In her letters she was often critical of Mrs Wardroper and felt that in some respects her judgement of character, her work and her training of the nurses could have been bettered. There is no indication that Mrs Wardroper was aware of this herself. Nevertheless, they generally collaborated well on issues of moral guardianship, at one point going to great lengths to decide as to whether or not to dismiss one young lady because she 'made eyes'. For the Nightingale probationer any flirtation could be punished by instant dismissal; evidently to become a nurse you had to leave such things behind. Although the probationer in question was seen as a competent woman, and her moral character was said to be unexceptionable, Mrs Wardroper wrote that she seemed unable to refrain from 'using her eyes unpleasantly', but before formal dismissal, should we consider whether she might grow out of it as she matures?'. To protect their moral welfare, and because of the area St Thomas's Hospital was located in, probationers were only allowed out in pairs, regardless of the inevitable fact that many would separate as soon as they turned the corner.

By the early 1870s, St Thomas's Hospital had increased considerably in size, and there was also a greater number of beds, which gave a great deal of extra work to Mrs Wardroper. The Nightingale Council advised that an assistant to the matron was now required. Mrs Wardroper objected because she felt that an assistant would come between her and her nurses. It was not until October 1872 that Miss Torrance, one of Florence Nightingale's stars, was appointed. Miss Torrance was described as one of the most capable Superintendents that St Thomas's Hospital had ever trained. She had previously worked at the Infirmary St Pancras, one of the first London hospitals to ask for a trained matron. Miss Torrance had taken with her nine nurses, setting up her own training scheme for pauper nurses in 1871. She had commenced at St Pancras in 1869 and during those two years, in the same way as all her colleagues, she faced many difficulties. One particular problem was the head nurses. They neither understood nor were capable of doing the training. Miss Torrance, however, proved more than a match for this, working closely with Dr Dowse, the medical officer. She eventually married Dr Dowse, much to the chagrin of Florence Nightingale. The effect this had on Miss Nightingale was profound; she described it as 'the greatest shock one ever had in one's life'.

Sadly by the autumn of 1873, Mrs Wardroper was starting to show signs of high stress levels. She would lose her temper with people, acting almost like a tyrant. Convinced that others were spying on her, she began to develop her own network, setting nurse against nurse and junior staff against senior staff. Mrs Wardroper was once accused by Nightingale of behaving like a 'semi-insane king', but at her best she had been inspirational. Mrs Wardroper finally retired in 1887, after being Superintendent of the Nightingale Training School for twenty-seven years. She was by then over seventy years of age.

Although great changes had been made, many sectors of nursing were still in a parlous state. This was reflected in a letter written in 1877 by 'Sister Casualty' at St Bartholomew's Hospital. She complained that drunkenness was very common among the staff nurses, who were chiefly lower-class women. They were still of bad character, with little or no education, and precious little knowledge of nursing. Many still had no experience of nursing even though they were engaged as staff nurses. One woman, she remembered, had been a lady's maid, and had never done a day's nursing. She was, however, of a better class than any of the others and at least respectable. It was still not unusual for friends of the patients to bring in presents of gin to bribe the nurses with in order that they would be kind to their friend. The worst women were those who used to come in to look after very bad cases, more particularly at night; she described them as dreadful people, possessing neither character nor ability.

A particular problem for the newly trained nurses became apparent when they went to other hospitals; they were often at odds with the matron in post. The matron could be a woman of low quality. The newly trained nurses presented a real threat to these matrons; in many cases the new nurses were women of a higher social class, and they could gain credibility from both doctors and patients through their leadership and skills, whereas the existing matron could only gain 'respect' through fear.

The Fund was constantly short of Superintendent Nurses

(matrons) of a high calibre, and Miss Nightingale constantly agonized over this. What she wanted to do was send to any hospital that requested, or wherever the opportunity arose, a small number of trained nurses and a trained matron. She was looking for, but found great difficulty in getting, the right sort of calibre nurse who had both authority and powers of orga- nization. The problem was compounded because prior to this time women had not thought to learn the necessary technical details about the hospital. Nightingale insisted that her matrons should have undisputed supremacy. Matron was to be responsible for the whole nursing staff; the nursing in the hospital; the kitchen, laundry and domestic staff; the nursing school, and for the appointment and dismissal of nursing staff. From the moment probationers entered to the time they left, they were to be under her authority. Her nurses were expected to be resident at the hospital for their social and moral good, and be of exemplary character. About these matters Florence Nightingale was adamant, and wherever 'her' trained nurses worked, a matron would be in place.

Many of the new matrons must have set out ill-equipped for the task ahead of them. They were relatively inexperienced with minimal training of one year or less. Hostility from the medical establishment, insanitary conditions and sexual innu- endoes from male patients were upsetting to many of these ladies. Trained at the relatively cosseted St Thomas's Hospital, they went to work in some of the most frightful environ- ments. In major cities conditions in hospitals could be appalling and worse, they were women taking lead roles in a male-dominated world. It is to the everlasting credit of these women that they so resolutely stuck to their task.

The new matron role immediately posed a challenge to the traditional power that the medical establishment had enjoyed; this was further heightened by the subsequent removal of nurses from the authority of the doctors. The conflict between doctors and matrons was not just a conflict between male and female authority (although many matrons were now women drawn from similar social backgrounds to the men and must have posed a great threat to them in this regard), it was also a conflict between one profession, medicine, which had recently secured its professional status, and nursing, itself looking for professional recognition. Doctors were not going to let them infiltrate their hard-won ground easily.

In finding their feet, the new matrons were highly territorial, often trying to outdo each other. In 1887 Florence Nightingale lamented, 'It is shocking how often there is a jealous, not friendly, rivalry between hospital matrons.' The relationship should have been based around a friendly network of mutual assistance (after all they had all come from the same training system), but was often based instead more on rivalry. Nightingale further complained of limited communication and association between the matrons, something that greatly disappointed her.

By 1880, a pattern was emerging where matrons were more clearly in authority over their nurses. Assistant matrons would directly support them. The Sister role was clearly defined as she was in charge at ward level, sometimes called the matron's 'lieutenant', a position of considerable responsibility. Reporting directly to matron, they would have entire charge of their ward. These sisters were crucial for developing clinical competence on the wards and for the future success of nurse training.

The day staff of nurses would normally comprise a sister in charge, a staff nurse and three probationers. The day nurses came on duty at 7 a.m. and went off duty at 9 p.m. with two hours free for meals. Any nursing lectures had to be attended during this time. 'Ward Maids' and 'Scrubbers' ostensibly supplemented the work of the nurses, but nurses were still expected to do domestic duties.

In 1872 the matter of matrons' training was raised officially. A letter was addressed to Lord Beauchamp from Henry Bonham Carter stating that 'the matron must be trained', otherwise matron would be responsible for the conduct of nurses and for placing them to the house surgeon, but the nurses would then have the surgeon not the matron as their superintendent. He thought that the whole female staff ought to be responsible to the matron or there would be a lack of moral discipline. The matron would see that the nurses carried out the orders of the medical men concerning the treatment of the patients. Any complaints against nurses by medical staff or patients would be made directly to the matron who, alone, should take action. Any complaint against the matron would, of course, be made to the committee.

It was not until the middle of the 1870s before training began to be requisite upon appointment for both the matron and the sister, although untrained matrons continued to be appointed even early in the twentieth century.

IV
Pioneers and Martyrs

The first Nightingale Matrons were often called superintendents of nurses, and they proved to be true pioneers facing enormous obstacles. They had to front a world dominated by men who were not ready to yield power over to them, but by 1857 more than fifty matrons had secured posts throughout Britain and the Commonwealth.

The Brownlow Infirmary, Liverpool, was one of the first hospitals outside London to request Nightingale nurses. Mr Rathbone, a Liverpool philanthropist, persuaded Miss Nightingale to send trained nurses, with Miss Agnes Jones as Superintendent.

Agnes Jones was born in 1832, the daughter of Colonel Jones of Londonderry and the niece of Sir John Lawrence. A well educated, deeply religious lady, Miss Nightingale wrote of her, 'Pretty and young, rich and witty, ideal in her beauty as a Louis XIV shepherdess'. Like Miss Nightingale, she commenced her nurse training at the Kaiserswerth Institute, Germany. In 1862 she was encouraged by Nightingale to complete her training for one year at St Thomas's School of Nursing. Entering in 1863, she was spoken of by Mrs Wardroper as being the best probationer they had ever had. Her record at the school states that she was 'trustworthy, methodical and highly qualified for a position where intelligence and energy are required'. In the superintendence of her nurses, her religious and moral influences were to prove most valuable.

The Infirmary was a dismal place and almost out of the control of those who ran it. To keep order, the police regularly had to patrol some of the wards. In 1866 Agnes Jones, along with twelve other nurses, was given the task of organizing the nursing service for the twelve hundred patients confined there. It was with some reluctance that Miss Jones accepted the post. It was also with some reluctance that Florence Nightingale allowed her to go. Miss Nightingale had considerable reservations about Miss Jones. She was anxious that Miss Jones, a deeply religious lady, might not know 'what sin and wickedness were'. She was, however, to find out quickly at the Infirmary.

Nothing could have prepared her for what she faced. The pauper patients were described as behaving worse than animals; vicious habits, ignorance and idiocy met her on every side; drunkenness was universal and staff were only considered drunk if they were incapable of standing. Immorality and filth were commonplace; the patients wore the same shirts for several weeks; bedding was only changed and washed once a month, and food was at starvation levels. The number of patients was very large, and when it rose occasionally to well over 1500, it was overwhelming. As usual there were administrative difficulties. Miss Jones's position and powers were not properly defined. The supply of food was by outside contract, over which she had little control. 'It is like Scutari over again,' Miss Nightingale lamented. To make matters worse, there were high levels of resistance to the 'hoity-toity' London nurses because the hospital was almost entirely run by pauper nurses. Although there were thirty-five dismissals within the first month, Miss Jones was instructed to re-train the remainder, which proved a failure. It was a year before she was able to dispense completely with their services.

Having only twelve nurses to organize the care for this large number of patients, the task was daunting. Certainly she found the work intimidating. The wards of the Infirmary were at one point likened to Dante's *Inferno*.[1] Sick children slept seven or eight to a bed. Even the older inmates faced similar conditions. Double beds in hospitals were not uncommon, nor were multiple sleeping arrangements unusual in working-class homes.

Miss Jones was not always given the full authority that she needed – she even had to ask permission from the governors to leave the hospital. But like Mrs Wardroper had done, she started one ward at a time, requisitioning new stock, improving catering facilities and introducing disciplined care. With constant support from Miss Nightingale she overcame many of the obstacles. Working under great pressure at the Infirmary however, sometimes working for as long as eighteen hours in one day, had taken its toll on her health. On 1 February 1869, Miss Jones wrote to Miss Nightingale that she had been ill; on 19 February she died of typhus contracted at the Infirmary. Florence Nightingale was devastated. In *Goodwords* June 1868, she wrote about her sadness at the death of this remarkable lady; that she had been a woman, attractive and rich, young and witty, yet veiled and silent, distinguished by genius. She wrote of how she had worked hard to train herself in order that she could train others, and how her faith had sustained her; that she 'over-worked because others under-work'. Miss Nightingale was determined that her death should not be in vain. So profound was her loss, that Agnes Jones became the inspiration for the central character of Miss Nightingale's eulogy, 'Una and the Lion' (1868).

On 7 November 1871, Miss Mary Barclay took over as Superintendent at the Royal Infirmary, Edinburgh. It was not the fine hospital it is now, and Miss Nightingale was no lover of the hospital, describing it as 'a "beast" of a place and a den of thieves'. Miss Nightingale thought Miss Barclay had simplicity, straightforwardness, uncompromising duty, ideas, strong will, courage and sense, but she had one reservation, that Barclay was a poor judge of character – a complaint Nightingale had about many of her nurses. She also described her as a splendid leader of women – first in everything – a mother to her nurses. The nurses sent to the Infirmary were older women, described as wiry, and strong on their legs and in their heads, absolutely trustworthy and having something of a missionary spirit, so Miss Barclay had to be more than a mother; she was the leader, and had to be of strong character.

The place was unrefined and disorderly, so much so that Miss Barclay immediately took great pains to ensure that the food and accommodation were improved and met the needs of the patients. The advantage of having a woman such as Miss Barclay in charge was that she 'carried the female nurses with her in everything'. Eventually, and to the credit of Miss Barclay, nurses trained at St Thomas's Hospital staffed all twenty-two wards at the Infirmary. Unfortunately, Miss Barclay appeared to be displaying the symptoms of strain. She had begun to share the night watch twice a fortnight and the long hours and responsibilities proved too much. Under this pressure of work her health deteriorated and she became unable to continue as Superintendent. She retired in January 1875 and continued to nurse throughout her retirement in Cornwall until her death in June 1895.

Miss Pringle was next to be appointed Superintendent of the Royal Infirmary, Edinburgh, early in 1874. She had arrived with the first party of nurses under Miss Barclay. Although she was reluctant initially, she proved to be an admirable successor to Miss Barclay. Known to Miss Nightingale as 'The Pearl', and to the training school as 'Sister Albert', Miss Angelique Lucille Pringle was one of the youngest pupils to enter St Thomas's Training School. Her report on completion of training stated that she was 'an active and intelligent practical nurse, particularly in the surgical department – a person of superior abilities and education, as is apparent from the manner of reporting her care and notes of lectures – both highly creditable'. Her years at Edinburgh were said to have been outstanding. Like Mrs Wardroper, she possessed great organizational skills, but unlike Mrs Wardroper she was never fully confident in her own abilities.

In 1887, following the retirement of Mrs Wardroper, Miss Pringle moved from Edinburgh to take the post of Matron at St Thomas's Hospital. In the same year, she was invited to attend a meeting of the newly formed Matrons' Committee of the Hospitals' Association. This was a completely new concept for matrons and provoked quite a reaction from no less a figure than Florence Nightingale. This was to be the first 'association' for nurses, and with Miss Manson (later Mrs Bedford Fenwick), Matron of St Bartholomew's Hospital, she formed the British Nurses' Association (from 1891, the Royal British Nurses' Association) at approximately the same time.

Within less than three years of taking over at St Thomas's Hospital, Miss Pringle had joined the Roman Catholic Church, thus causing an instant conflict between her desire to remain in the post and Miss Nightingale's conviction that the Protestant committee would oppose it. Miss Pringle therefore reluctantly tendered her resignation in early 1890 which nevertheless still caused Miss Nightingale great distress. Miss Pringle was later to become noted for her pioneering work in the workhouse infirmaries of Ireland and America.

Miss Louisa McKay Gordon was the next Matron appointed to St Thomas's Hospital. She had been Assistant at the Royal Infirmary, Liverpool, for four years and Matron of the General Infirmary, Leeds, since 1874. Miss Gordon was an entirely different person in character and temperament from Miss Pringle. She was appointed in February 1890 and remained Superintendent for twelve years.

In September 1861, a portion of the Nightingale Fund was used to start a midwives' school at King's College Hospital where Miss Mary Jones was Matron. Miss Jones had kept in close contact with Miss Nightingale. Many letters were passed between the two of them reflecting this close relationship. In one of their letters Miss Nightingale questioned the age range of nurses proposed at King's College. She had no problem with the lower starting age of twenty-five, but was most bemused by the upper limit of forty. She asked 'Do you not find it difficult to teach a woman of near 40 anything like nursing, if she has not begun before?' On the other hand Miss Nightingale objected to the idea of refusing to admit deserted wives; she thought this was rather hard.

Mary Cadbury was born in 1839 in Birmingham. Her father was a draper and the family can be traced back to the twelfth century. Both her parents were involved with caring for the sick, in particular her mother was said to be most skilled in nursing care. Following their example, Miss Cadbury's interest in nursing grew and she devoted more and more time to the sick and infirm. As if in natural consequence, in 1873 she entered the training school of St Thomas's Hospital, London, where she proved to be one of the most able pupils. She then began work at the Highgate Workhouse Infirmary before further training at the District Nursing Home in Bloomsbury under the leadership of Mrs Craven, and then she spent two and a half years at Whalley Range, Manchester, as a District Nurse. Miss Cadbury was appointed Lady Superintendent at the Liverpool Parish Infirmary. Her first appointment as a matron was at West Street, Sheffield, and later she was to become Matron at the Queen's Hospital, Birmingham, in 1890. Throughout this time she continued to correspond with Miss Nightingale.

At Birmingham, Miss Cadbury proved to be outstanding and an excellent ambassador for the Nightingale training system. Having written in 1873 that she was entirely absorbed in the 'outwardness' of her patients, throughout her career she continued her emphasis on the physical cure of patients. Only later did she combine this with her religious beliefs, particularly for comforting the dying. Miss Cadbury died while still in her post in 1896.

In Dublin, Ireland, the new Adelaide Hospital was opened in 1858 (the first Adelaide had been opened in 1839). Miss Bramwell was appointed Lady Superintendent that same year, her post commencing on the 21 August. Recommended by Miss Nightingale, Miss Bramwell had been one of the successful nurses at Scutari in the Crimea. Only in the post for eight months, her work received a glowing report from the hospital Annual General Meeting. 'Her experience in regulating and superintending hospitals, and especially in training nurses, and directing "nursetending" in general, it is trusted will be found most beneficial.' During her time she established the basis for future nurse training. Mrs Ruttle succeeded Miss Bramwell in 1859. Having no formal training, she went to the Kaiserswerth Institute in Germany, as Miss Nightingale had done. Following four weeks' training, she returned and set up a successful one-year training course for nurses. She retired in 1872.

By the turn of the century, every major hospital in Britain had a Matron or Lady Superintendent of Nursing. Nurses and matrons were wanted throughout the Commonwealth, and in America. Of the Australian contingent, Miss Lucy Osburn was appointed Matron of the Sydney Royal Infirmary.

Miss Osburn entered nurse training as a pupil at St Thomas's at the age of twenty-nine and was described at the time as being a lady of superior birth and mistress of several languages. Miss Osburn and her group of four nurses arrived at the Sydney Infirmary in March 1868. The staffing consisted of twenty-three males and five females drawn largely from the reformed convict population. Transportation of convicts had ceased twenty years previously. The management system was chaotic, and the conditions were horrendous; vermin, lack of water and poor sanitation were rife, and there was a general lack of compassion too. Patients were left to lie in soiled beds, unwashed and unattended, with the excuse that the doctor had said they were not to be disturbed.[2] Many other things too did not bode well for these nurses.

Miss Osburn expected to take charge as Matron in the Sydney Infirmary, but the staff objected. The very idea of a woman being in charge was anathema to the Australian nursing and medical staff. They were not used to such a thing, and certainly did not expect a woman to arrive and take over as leader of nursing. Indeed the management saw no merit at all in having females do the nursing.[3] They believed that formal, and even informal, training was a waste of time and that these educated women would only cause further trouble. The conditions now facing Miss Osburn and her nurses were as appalling as the conditions at Scutari and Liverpool.

Miss Nightingale's confidence in Miss Osburn was shattered as a result of a letter indiscretion in which Osburn 'gossiped' about her voyage, and about a Duke, also a passenger. A relative had the letter printed and circulated and it was nearly Miss Osburn's undoing. Miss Nightingale wrote to her cousin, Henry Bonham-Carter (who was also Secretary to the Nightingale Fund from 1861 to 1914), that the 'goose of a man' had printed the information for private distribution. Miss Nightingale was furious. Her brother-in-law, Sir Harry Verney MP, a 'persuasive sort of person & also firm in his purpose', went to the gentleman to explain the scandal if the letter reached the newspapers, the Queen or the Colonial Office. 'Nothing could exceed his fright & annoyance – at what he had done. And he instantly consented to withdraw the copies[4].

At the end of the three-year contract Miss Nightingale wrote to Henry Bonham-Carter expressing concerns about Miss Osburn's abilities. However, she not only succeeded at the Sydney Hospital but she established there the base for successful nurse training throughout Australia. Linda Bolland, Project Director, Queensland, Australia, suggests that Miss Osburn is greatly respected even to this day. Miss Osburn's influence was also responsible for some similarities between the roles of matrons in Australia and in Britain. Mrs Bolland found herself still being called 'Matron' in the 1990s. (Unfortunately the stereotyping of matron as a 'dragon' is just as familiar there as here.)

Mary Barker was one of the nurses who accompanied Miss Osburn. She became a future matron at Edinburgh and could be described as a woman dedicated to her work. She applied herself to nursing with great vigour and diligence, but with little sense of humour. Shortly after arriving in Sydney, Miss Osburn wrote that most of Miss Barker's work had been in a male accident ward. Here difficulties and trials arose, such as rarely occur in a general surgical ward or medical ward. In male accident wards, nurses had to act with much promptness and deal with men who were usually of the roughest and most depraved sort. 'Miss Barker's temperament, not naturally amiable, has not grown more so. She is, however, a good nurse and her patients will never suffer from neglect.'

Miss Barker, as was the habit with Nightingale nurses, also wrote to Miss Nightingale, this time about the conditions existing at the Sydney Infirmary in 1868. She described the wards as rough and dirty; there were dirty skirts and gowns hanging everywhere; the nurses were dressed in old skirts and jackets of all colours and did not wear caps. She thought that the scrubbers at St Thomas's Hospital were of a more respectable class. The ventilation was poor; patients could be left in bed for weeks without having had their hands and faces washed; when the nurse had to wash the patients before placing them in clean beds, the old bed would be found to have practically rotted away. The so-called nurses had accepted bedsores and vermin as perfectly natural. Rags were frequently patched together to make bedding and it was not unusual for nursing staff to tear up bed sheets to make poultices or cleaning rags. No wonder Miss Osburn and her group with their spotless nurses' uniforms were so greatly admired.

On return to England in 1873, Miss Barker took an appointment at the Royal Edinburgh Infirmary where Miss Pringle was still Matron. Miss Barker was eventually appointed Matron of the Edinburgh Convalescent Home on the recommendation of Miss Pringle, but either the Sydney experience had proven too severe, or she was not able to make a satisfactory transition to the role of Matron, because in any event, she was sadly admitted to the Prestwich Asylum where she died on 4 December 1889.

The other four nurses who accompanied Miss Osburn took up places in other parts of Australia as hospital matrons; Miss Turriff led the way with her appointment as Matron of the new Alfred Hospital in Melbourne, Victoria.

Miss Alice Fisher was born in England on 14 June 1839. Her father was the Revd George Fisher. He did not enjoy good health and, after a long illness, was nursed by Miss Fisher until his death. It was during this time that she made up her mind to care for the sick. Following his death she commenced training at St Thomas's Hospital, London. A great success at the school and an able organizer, Miss Fisher was appointed Assistant Superintendent at the Royal Infirmary, Edinburgh. She was then appointed Assistant Superintendent at the Fever Hospital, Newcastle, and Addenbroke's Hospital, Cambridge. She was then appointed superintendent at the General Hospital, Birmingham, where she was noted for the introduction of nurse training.

Being an undoubted leader in nursing, in 1884 Alice Fisher was encouraged to take the post at Superintendent at the Philadelphia Hospital, Blockley, in the United States. Here she faced a similar experience to that of the great workhouses in Britain. The many hundred patients were being nursed by other inmates who themselves had been detailed to look after the sick. Miss Fisher had learned her skills well, however, and with her able assistant Miss Hornor, set about reforming the hospital and introducing training. The School of Nurses of the Philadelphia Hospital was recognized for, and still is an outstanding example of, the indomitable courage of this woman. Her organization skills were also felt throughout Philadelphia, where she supported the reorganization of many other hospitals. Miss Fisher was a remarkable woman who set aside her own health problems, a heart condition diagnosed at St Thomas's Hospital while in training, to develop nursing as a highly respected occupation. Although America did not follow the Nightingale pattern of a matron as head of nursing, Miss Fisher is still remembered as a pioneer of nurse training. She died on 3 June 1888.

Maria Machin began her nursing career at the Nightingale School in 1872 as a Lady Probationer. Miss Nightingale saw her as a woman of great capacity in mind and body but susceptible to the strains and stresses of hospital life. One incident (a septic finger) necessitated Maria being almost 'laid up' and protected from dusting and washing for some time. She was, nevertheless, seen to be a potential leader of nurses. In 1875 she left with four head nurses to join the staff of Montreal General Hospital, Canada. Her task was to set up a training school on the principles of St Thomas's Hospital. Initially she wrote of her high hopes and successes, appearing confident in her abilities; however the authorities were antagonistic to the scheme and the construction of the promised hospital and nurses' home had not begun. After two years the letters were more doubtful and lacked the conviction she needed to continue the reforms: 'I am getting to think the range of my superintending duties is too extensive for me ... I often wish I were a ward sister instead of superintendent, I'm so much happier nursing the sick than governing the ones who are well.' By 1877 the committee investigating rising costs at the Montreal General reported that she had been extravagant, over-ordering food and exercising inadequate control. She returned to England the following year and was given the post of Matron at St Bartholomew's on Miss Nightingale's request.

By the turn of the century matrons were establishing themselves in most hospitals and nursing was beginning to gain some real status. Having worked so hard, matrons were determined that the 'dark age' of nursing was to become history. Matrons had gone about their work with a great deal of disciplinary zeal. They were singularly responsible for enhancing nursing standards in the hospitals and for promoting the respectability of women working as nurses. The gains they had achieved were considerable and this was not only in nursing. Women were forging a significant place in society. The movement for the emancipation of women was making progress with the Women's Social and Political Union founded in Manchester by Emmeline Pankhurst in 1903. It could be argued that the advent of the modern matron and the role women played in the First World War influenced the decision on women's suffrage.

The twentieth century began with ambitious initiatives for the expansion and upgrade of many hospitals. Electric lighting began to replace gas lighting and the telephone became an essential tool of communication. X-ray, discovered in 1895 by W. Roenteg, began to change the way diagnoses were made. Cross-infection was more fully understood and the main protection was scrupulous cleanliness. Early in the new century, after Queen Victoria had died, a number of new hospitals were built in commemoration of her. Unfortunately, many hospitals still remained places to avoid; the wealthy employed their own private nurses, with the poor generally occupying the hospital beds. Health problems were mainly associated with infectious diseases. Tuberculosis was rife, venereal disease rampant, and occupational injuries were depleting the workforce. Some of the poor house infirmaries were still in a deplorable state, along with many of the voluntary and fever hospitals. The infirmaries catered for a larger number of patients namely the chronically sick and those with little ability to pay, with the voluntary hospitals providing for the more acute patients who could pay a contribution to their care. The quality of matrons in these establishments varied greatly, but with the increasing numbers of trained nurses, the position was changing.

In the larger hospitals in both London and the provinces, the title of Matron was not always used. Miss Florence M. Calvert took the title Lady Superintendent of Nurses instead of Matron at the Manchester Royal Infirmary, from 1891 to 1907. Miss M.E. Sparshott, CBE, also kept the title Lady Superintendent until her retirement in 1929. Matrons of this time could be called the most fiercely autocratic group of all periods of nursing. They had gained strong positions in the hospitals and were using them. Women of strength and character, such as Sarah Swift of Guy's Hospital, Miss Hamilton of University College Hospital, and Miss Lückes at the London Hospital, were determined nursing should never return to the Sarah Gamp image again.

The rules relating to matrons at the University College Hospital (UCH), London, reflected these changes. Opened in 1834, the hospital had a history of appointing high-quality matrons, and Miss Harriet E. Hamilton, appointed in 1899 following an extensive rebuilding programme, was no exception. A Nightingale-trained nurse, it was to be her task to re-staff the hospital and form a new training school. Miss Hamilton commenced at a salary of £125 with new rules of work brought out the same year. These were:

- Matron shall be single or widowed, not below thirty or above forty-five years of age, and must reside in the hospital.
- She shall appoint the nurses, probationers, lady probationers, and female servants, and a certain number of ward maids.

- Select the sisters and recommend them for appointment to the Nursing Committee.
- She shall maintain the authorized staff of well-trained sisters and nurses and supply such extra nurses as shall from time to time be required.
- She shall be responsible for:
  The complete training of every nurse in every department of the hospital.
  The proper fulfilment of their duties by the female staff.
  The daily diet orders for the patients, and the orders for provisions and all other articles required in the Nursing Department.
- She shall visit each ward of the hospital at least once every day, and shall see that everything within her department is kept clean and in good order.

Reports of Miss Hamilton were glowing, describing a gentle, cheerful and good-humoured lady. Miss Hamilton's time at UCH was not easy and reflects a period when matrons were still having to fight to maintain standards, at a time when funds were scarce throughout London and provincial hospitals. Her great success at UCH was the establishment of the nurse training unit, and it was no surprise when, after three years, she was appointed Matron of St Thomas's Hospital.

Miss Dora Finch was the next matron at UCH and remained in the post for twenty-one years. Very different from Miss Hamilton, she preferred to be less visible. Seeming somewhat austere, she was dignified and self-effacing. Her time as matron was noted for an improvement in the calibre of nurses entering the hospital training school.

Nursing was still in a state of chaos with no central figure of authority. On the one hand, Miss Nightingale was opposed to any form of nurse registration and on the other, Miss Ethel Gordon Manson was striving to gain registration for nurses. Born on 26 January 1857, Miss Manson was the daughter of a wealthy doctor. Whilst still only in her teens, Miss Manson became a paying probationer at the Children's Hospital, Nottingham. She then went to the Royal Infirmary, Manchester, to complete her nurse training. Twenty years later, now Mrs Bedford Fenwick, she recalled her first 'interview' with matron. She presented matron with 'an offering of great odorous Czar violets'. A few words sufficed to express Miss Manson's desire to commence nursing. 'I offered ten stones of perfect physical development, youth, and boundless enthusiasm, she thought the offer sound.' And they struck a bargain then and there.

Remarkable in her speed of promotion, at the age of twenty-one, having experienced previous rejections at many hospitals for being too young even to train, she was now a Ward Sister at the London Hospital. The next step for this amazing lady was in 1881 when St Bartholomew's Hospital required a new matron. Miss Manson confidently put in a personal appearance at the hospital, and despite her age of twenty-four, was appointed Matron. But at the age of thirty, in 1887, she married Dr Bedford Fenwick and retired from active nursing; Miss Nightingale was devastated. Her contribution at St Bartholomew's, and her subsequent contribution to the development of nursing as a profession, was unique. By the time she resigned, the school of nursing had introduced a three-year course, had national renown, and a certificate from the hospital was highly valued. Working conditions for nurses had improved with a cut in hours and far better quality food.

In 1887, Mrs Bedford Fenwick founded the British Nursing Association and became its permanent president. In 1894 she formed the Matrons' Council of Great Britain and Ireland for those matrons who wanted state registration. Now she could concentrate on her other important work, the introduction of nurse registration. She believed that registration would largely abolish 'bad nurses'. Against a background of resistance it took Mrs Fenwick twenty-nine years (until 1916) to succeed. The Articles of Association were drawn up and the College of Nursing Limited opened on 27 March 1916.

The principle objectives of the College were:

1. To promote the better education and training of nurses and the advancement of nursing as a profession in all or any of its branches.

2. To promote uniformity of curriculum.
3. To recognize approved nursing schools.
4. To make and maintain a register of persons to whom certificates of proficiency or of training and proficiency have been granted.
5. To promote Bills in Parliament for any objective connected with the interests of the nursing profession and, in particular, with nurse education, organization, protection, or for their recognition by the state.

Three broad categories of nurse were to be covered for registration. They were the existing nurses who had been engaged in 'bona fide' (good faith or good intentions) practice; nurses who completed their training after registration but before the new entrance scheme was properly instituted; and future trainees who would qualify by passing the appropriate professional examinations. Midwives would have on their door 'By Examination' to differentiate them from the 'bona fide' midwife.

Isla Stewart followed Miss Ethel Manson at St Bartholomew's Hospital and was Matron from 1887-1910. She was the first President of the Matrons' Council working closely with Mrs Fenwick. Stewart was born in Scotland and was another lady who had a remarkable beginning to her career in nursing. She was only nine months into her training as a pupil nurse when she was appointed Ward Sister at St Thomas's Hospital. After two matron posts at small hospitals, she applied for, and gained, the appointment of Matron of St Bartholomew's Hospital at the age of thirty. She was an energetic commanding figure with great presence.

By this time, nurses were being revered as had never happened before. Miss Stewart, by no means a sentimentalist, brought the nurses back down to earth. She wrote that the pedestal that nurses occupied in the eyes of many people was a purely imaginary one. It had been the fashion to speak and think of a nurse's life as 'a beautiful renunciation of the world and worldly pleasures, the devotion of a life to soothing the dying and consoling the living'. She believed that this was a mistake, and that self-sacrifice was not a leading characteristic. Nurses, she wrote, were hard-working women who, as a rule, slept soundly and ate heartily. A nurse's position, she thought, was that of a woman wishing for independence, owing no man anything and wishing for no undeserved praise or blame. Her position towards the hospital was purely commercial, receiving board, lodging and a small salary in return for work done. A nurse's position towards her patients she viewed as practically that of an attendant paid by the hospital, to wait upon the patients, and to do everything in her power for their comfort and well-being. Nurses to Miss Stewart were simply working women, bound to give their best efforts to the institution that paid them for their work.[5]

Trained at the Middlesex Hospital, Miss Lückes was appointed Matron of the London Hospital, Whitechapel, in 1880, following the resignation of Miss Swift, who had been the matron from 1878. Within no time at all, Miss Lückes, an intimate friend of Miss Nightingale's, attended the house committee meeting to tell them that the nursing staff at the London Hospital was grossly inadequate both in quality and quantity. She introduced a two-year course at a time when others were instituting three-year courses. This in turn brought her into conflict with Mrs Bedford Fenwick and even resulted in her being called before a Parliamentary Select Committee, but Miss Lückes won the day. She was eventually one of the first matrons in England to open a Preliminary Training School, in 1895.

During Miss Lückes's time at the London Hospital, many nurses were employed as private nurses. Mainly middle-class patients, who were treated in their own homes, employed these nurses. It was an important source of income to the hospital. In this role a nurse could travel anywhere in the country and be nursing illnesses such as cancer or gout or eye problems. Miss Lückes was a believer in keeping in close touch with her nurses as she thought that this both created a loyalty to the hospital and also a desire to do the hospital credit. Known as the 'Maker of Matrons' because so many of her nurses became matrons, Miss Lückes was awarded the

Royal Red Cross and the CBE in 1917. She died in February 1919, soon after being awarded the Lady of Grace Order of St John.

When the First World War broke out in August 1914, it was to change the lives of everyone. For women it meant separation, role change and new learning. Many could still not read or write, but now there were forms to fill in for allowances, separation (if married) or child allowances (if single). A whole new world opened to them, with opportunities to work in factories or in sectors such as the Voluntary Aid Detachment (VAD). The VADs were a voluntary group of women who would man the hospitals at home and abroad. There was great resistance to them from the trained nursing staff, who deeply resented their presence and saw them as a threat to registration and were concerned that these untrained nurses would take their jobs. They had no reason to worry since very few continued in hospital life after the war ended.

Throughout nursing history there have been many nurse heroines. One nurse who symbolized the spirit of sacrifice for others during the First World War was Edith Cavell. Edith Cavell was born on 4 December 1865 at Swarsdeston, Norfolk. Her first experience of nursing was as governess to the four children of a Brussels lawyer. She had to return to England when her father fell ill, but on his recovery and at the age of thirty, she decided to make nursing her career. She applied to the London Hospital, Whitechapel for nurse training, and was interviewed and accepted by Matron, Miss Eva Lückes. On completion of her training, Miss Cavell took the post of Night Superintendent at the St Pancras Infirmary, London. St Pancras was in the process of changing from a poor law workhouse infirmary to a medical institution. From this post she then moved to being Assistant Matron at Shoreditch Infirmary. After a further move to Manchester as Assistant Matron, she was offered the post of Matron of the Berkendael Institute training school in Brussels. By 1908, Belgian hospitals were substituting English-trained nurses for their nuns, a change which can be attributed almost exclusively to Miss Cavell.

As an English nurse in Belgium at the start of the First World War, Edith Cavell found herself uniquely placed to help Allied servicemen. Shortly after the German occupation of Brussels, she found herself deeply involved in the escape of British soldiers. Two wounded soldiers required urgent treatment and Miss Cavell did not hesitate to offer them refuge. From this point on, she was inextricably involved in the smuggling of more than two hundred soldiers across the Dutch border under cover of night. Inevitably, by spring 1915, the Germans were becoming suspicious of her activities. On 20 June, the Institute in the Rue de la Culture was inspected. Miss Cavell survived this initial inspection, but was arrested on the inspectors' return on 5 August. It is not known how a confession was obtained from her while she was in prison, but a lengthy confession was sufficient for her to be sent for trial. The trial began on 6 October 1915 and the death penalty was the inevitable outcome. Her last letter was to her beloved nurses. Edith Cavell was shot in the execution ground in Brussels on 12 October 1915. As a patriotic English woman, she represented the finest for selflessness and bravery. As a British nurse she represented all that was outstanding in nurse training and discipline.

Notes

1 There is some debate about the extent of the appalling conditions. An edition of the *Porcupine* (a Liverpool newspaper) from 1871 suggests some of the stories about the workhouse could be exaggerated.
2 Russell, L., 'Training Nurses at the Lucy Osburn School of Nursing' (*Education Enquiry*, vol. 2, 1979), pp. 35-54.
3 Anderson, M., 'The Women's Movement' in M. Atkinson (ed.) *Australia: Economic and Political Studies* (Macmillan, 1920), p. 284.
4 Vicinus, M., and Nergaard, B. (eds.), *Ever Yours, Florence Nightingale* (Virago Press, London, 1989).
5 Stewart, I., *Practical View of Nursing* (1890), pp. 162-163.

V
The Charming Irish Girl

Almost all modern matrons lived through one or both of the World Wars. Miss Emily MacManus was no exception. Through these two World Wars, Miss MacManus was instrumental in advancing nursing from its rigid Victorian roots to becoming a modern, professional nursing service.

Emily E.P. MacManus was born on 18 April 1886. To be born into a middle-class family in the nineteenth century, as Emily MacManus was, often meant enjoying enhanced privileges, privileges denied to the working class. Middle-class children had access to private education, often travelling abroad to finishing schools; they had more time for leisure pursuits; they were used to servants; however, this did not give automatic entry to daughters of the middle classes into universities, the study of medicine, or the military services. Any woman who wanted to be successful had to fight hard. They were encouraged to work yet few doors were open to them. Some women made it through university or medical school, but these were still the minority. Men had the right to vote but there was scant regard for women's political or legal rights. Self-determination for a daughter and equal rights for women were often at odds, but this social climate created many women who would not be held back, women who were not prepared to hide behind any amount of privilege. One such woman was Emily MacManus, the sort of woman we are unlikely to see the likes of again.

Her extensive family background (half-Irish, half-English) stretched way back to the days of Elizabeth I. One great-grandparent, Patrick MacManus, was a farmer, and her other great-grandparent was Leonard Strong, a sugar-plantation manager. Leonard Strong's family could boast the friendship of Admiral Nelson. Emily MacManus was born in Wandsworth and spent her childhood in Battersea. Her father was a much-loved local doctor who worked amongst the poor and social outcasts.. Her formal education was completed at the age of seventeen when she became her aunt's companion for a year. To encourage her social development, her parents arranged for her to live in the superintendent's house at Guy's Hospital for four years; her uncle was superintendent of the hospital.

For a young woman there were limited options available to her when choosing a worthwhile occupation. Nursing was by now a more respected vocation than it had been previously, and one in which an intelligent, enthusiastic, dedicated and independent young woman could advance herself. Miss MacManus had been steered towards the medical profession since childhood, with father, uncles and aunts all forging various successful careers. With the support of her uncle and matron Miss Sarah Smith, whom she knew well, Emily MacManus was appointed to be a nurse probationer at Guy's Hospital aged twenty-two, a year younger than was usual. Thus she started her nursing career, following in the hallowed family footsteps.

Her accommodation was basic, her room containing merely a bed, table and chair. There was a fixed wash-basin, a wardrobe, dressing table and a small rug. Though austere, it was better equipped than rooms provided in other hospitals, and almost luxurious in comparison to the conditions experienced by previous Guy's nurses. These older nurses would tell stories of living in the attic spaces above the wards with barely adequate gas lighting and little else. Their rations were so meagre they had to buy extra food to supplement the diet, cooking precariously over gaslight flames. Emily MacManus considered herself very fortunate.

The preliminary training for probationers lasted six weeks. During this time they were taught elementary anatomy, physiology, hygiene, invalid cookery, practical nursing procedures and nursing ethics. Emily MacManus, moved by the notion of ethical nursing, felt that the ethics lectures guided her throughout her life, as did the Nightingale maxim 'Difficulties are made to be overcome'. After just six weeks of theory, the junior probationers entered the wards for the first time, putting into practice what they had learned under the strict and watchful eye of Miss Swift. Trained in the nineteenth century, she believed that the ability to take responsibility was central to nurse leadership, a lesson Emily MacManus learned well. At the end of a two-month trial period Emily MacManus was allowed to sign her contract, agreeing to abide by the moral standards of Guy's, and willingly shouldering the mantle of responsibility which was seen as one of the principal virtues of a nurse.

As Emily MacManus progressed to senior probationer, she also took on increasing responsibility. Working in Guy's outpatients department, the largest and most comprehensive outpatients department in London, she gained invaluable experience, which would serve her well for future appointments. By the time she reached third-year status, she held the title of Head Nurse and, by 1912, her life as a nurse in training was over. On receipt of her certificate, she immediately arranged to take additional training as a midwife, not at Guy's, but at the East End Mother's Home in Commercial Road, Whitechapel. The matron at the maternity hospital, Margaret Anderson, was a formidable woman of the Florence Nightingale ilk. She demanded and ensured a high quality of work from the sister-midwives who acted as tutors and, as a consequence, the standard of education for students was superb.

Emily MacManus spent the next two years in Egypt, where she worked at the Kasr-el-Aini, a government hospital in Cairo. She was allotted a ward of her own and was the Sister-in-Charge of the men's medical section. On her return from Egypt, she was offered a temporary appointment at Guy's

Hospital as a relief duty sister. Her first post was that of second (junior) sister in the preliminary training school, where she taught hygiene and helped supervise practical classes in bandaging, bed-making, and surgical and medical procedures. She was then drafted to the post of relief lady-superintendent of the laundry-maids' hostel. The big steam laundry at Guy's was manned by laundry-maids who were – to use the language of the day – 'fallen girls', and the hospital served as their residential rescue home.

Miss MacManus took her first regular post in April 1914, as Sister in one of the accident wards at Guy's Hospital. At twenty-eight years of age, done in only four years, this was rapid progress for a nurse in such a prestigious hospital as Guy's. By the spring of the following year, her life was to change dramatically. As war casualties began to arrive from the battlefields of France, she decided to 'join up' in July 1915 as a Civil Nursing Reserve Sister. She was soon to leave for France.

She was sent to the 18th General Hospital at Etaples, where she stayed in the 'hutted' hospitals, working under highly experienced 'war veteran' sisters. She then moved on to Camiers with Matron Miss Minns, along with three regular army sisters. Within a year she was moved from her surgical marquee and was appointed Home Sister and Mess Sister, taking responsibility for the dietary requirements of all patients and staff. Initially life was hard, as it was for all the reserves. Insecurity on the part of the longer-serving staff brought a deep suspicion of new people. They were generally given the more menial tasks until they 'proved' themselves. This insecurity was heightened when VADs were introduced. The regulars were extremely jealous of these two groups and saw them as threatening their status quo. There had been a thirty-year battle for nurse registration and both groups were regarded as obstacles to put back the likelihood of success for the military nursing service.

In spite of herself Emily MacManus began to enjoy her job and, under matron's guidance, felt she was learning something new every day. She even learned how to butcher sheep and invent interesting dishes from rations of hard tack, bully-beef and cheese, a far cry from her genteel beginnings. At Christmas 1917, the American military hospitals arrived and took over various established hospitals in France. Miss Minns was drafted to Dieppe, to prepare a hotel on the beach as a Convalescence Home for Officers. Emily MacManus went with her as her assistant; this was a vast improvement on two years spent in flapping tents, dust and muddy fields. It was a significant step in her career.

The hotel could accommodate two hundred officers. A second hotel was taken and it boasted a surgeon's room, treatment room, staff quarters and a dining room. Many of the officers, young and old, were dazed and exhausted after their grim experiences and horrific injuries. They recovered slowly from their wounds and even more slowly from their psychological traumas. As the war grew worse, Emily MacManus was appointed to a temporary position outside Rouen. She was on night duty in charge of two, fifty-bed huts for fractures of limbs. To manage this she had only two nursing orderlies and a raw 'runner'.

Now only just in her thirties, having already seen so much suffering and pain, she was embroiled in war zone nursing. Faced with having to treat men with the most appalling injuries, she had to call on her reserves of self-discipline, selflessness, poise, compassion and personal bravery. The war did prove to be an extraordinary training ground, and for Emily MacManus a series of traumatic events through which she fought to survive. She, along with other nurses, worked day and night, with the deafening sound of heavy gunfire a constant reminder of more injured men yet to come, but she had inherited an inner strength and this served her well, helping her to find courage in the face of great adversity.

Enforced evacuation from Rouen mortified Emily MacManus. Leaving the wounded behind, she had never felt more sad or ashamed in her life. The extent of this human tragedy overwhelmed but also empowered her. At her new reserve field station, she stoically worked through the nights, assisting emergency operations often having to overcome her own terror in order to help save lives. Death stalked her during these terrible years. Tantalizingly close, it became a familiar companion. Living and working in extreme danger was accepted as a matter of realistic fact. Emily MacManus risked her own life many times – on one occasion she crawled amongst hundreds of gas victims, trying to save their sight before she, too, succumbed to the poison gas still leaking from their clothing. On another occasion she ran through an air raid to retrieve an urgently needed hypodermic needle whilst bombs exploded all around her. She gained the comparative safety of her room when there was an enormous explosion in the next street. As she ran back down the stairs another explosion occurred, nearer to the house. At that moment she bumped into a khaki-clad figure coming up the stairs. They clung together for a long minute, not saying a word. Then he went up and she continued her way down. Rough khaki and a kilt was all she knew about him, but he was a tower of strength to her at that moment.

By this stage of the war, these valiant women had no possessions but the clothes they stood up in. Moving from camp to camp they experienced the worst effects of warfare. They were an exhausted and destitute band, but they were not dispirited. Having experienced life in tents, being coated in mud, having to move at no notice; having witnessed gassing, mutilation and shell-shock, news of the armistice was welcome indeed. Word spread quickly, the sword of Damocles had been lifted, and a sense of relief swept through the whole camp, but this was swiftly to be followed by disaster as, once again, fate dealt a crippling blow. An influenza epidemic reached them, and patients went down like flies. Few of the injured men had reserves sufficient to fight this new illness. Emily MacManus described them as going under and dying with a swiftness as though they had black cholera. The epidemic wiped out many of the individuals she had fought so hard to save, a stark reminder of the frailty of life.

As if she had not suffered enough pain, Emily MacManus received news from England that her mother was desperately ill with pneumonia. Miss Minns moved quickly and Emily was put on the next boat for England. Still a young woman, Emily MacManus had acquired a reputation for courage, competence and fortitude. It was no surprise when in 1919 she received an invitation from Miss Margaret Hogg, who had succeeded Miss Haughton as Matron of Guy's, to return to her old hospital as assistant matron. She worked in this position for three and a half years. As was customary, her quarters were in the nurses' home where she had a first-class maid to wait on her.

For the first few months she found life at Guy's utterly intolerable. The past three and a half years had been spent in the open air under canvas. She had lived in a world of men; sick men, convalescent men, orderlies, officers, and men from every part of the commonwealth. All had talked about their jobs, about home, about life in general. All had accepted her as a comrade and most had been dependent on her. She had lived through their battles with them, learned to regard them as individuals rather than as 'superiors'. She had equal status within a world at war, a status which had no parallel in normal society now. She was plunged back into a world of women: student nurses, domestics, cleaners, ward sisters and office staff. It was a world of controlling forces and conflicting hierarchies, with male physicians and a female nursing strata. Although she was fully occupied arranging the nurses' work, assisting the matron, making her rounds, and sorting out the troubles and difficulties of a staff of a thousand women, she felt stifled and unreasonably restricted. Her movements were tightly controlled and she could only leave the hospital at stated hours. She was now restricted to a half-day's leave in the middle of the week, a weekend off once a fortnight, and she worked hours that stretched until eight at night. Despite holding wide powers as assistant matron, she felt that this power was not sufficient compensation for what she had lost – she had lost her freedom. Life had changed forever. She, like many young women, found it difficult to return to the pre-war world of social control, manifest within society and the medical profession.

The suffragist movement started as early as the 1860s, but

had only made slow progress by the turn of the century. However, the war and the new suffragette activists caused a new surge of activity in the struggle for both liberty and the right of women to vote. Realizing they could not count on political parties or organized labour movements, women found they had to do their own fighting for equality and justice. Non-activists of the calibre of Emily MacManus, through their own examples of determination and leadership, did a great deal towards bringing about success for the suffragist movement by 1930.

At Guy's Hospital, the usual tenure of the post of assistant matron was limited to three years. The post was generally regarded as the 'jumping-off' point for a matronship. Not ready for a life as confined and austere as that of a matron, Emily MacManus took a year out, and spent the time working alongside a 'children's physician' at the Dr Barnardo's Boys' Garden City. Together they conducted a series of experiments into the influence of diet on child growth and development. When the year was over she was once again encouraged to apply for the post of Matron. On this occasion, the editor of the *Nursing Times* wrote to her, sending particulars of a vacancy at the Bristol Royal Infirmary – one of the oldest voluntary hospitals in the west of England. She was appointed and took up the post a month later. She spent a very happy time working in Bristol, gaining a lot of experience in committee work, remaining there for three and a half years.

In 1927 MacManus received a letter from Herbert Eason, Superintendent of Guy's, encouraging her to apply for the post of Matron. Again she was successful. As Matron of Guy's Hospital, she managed a staff of eight hundred, and cared for a patient group numbering seven hundred. She had her own residence, which faced the Superintendent's House where she had spent many of her earlier years. Matron Emily MacManus had now taken on a more managerial role. Every week she would meet with the House Committee chaired by a Governor of the Bank of England. She would read the nominal roll, that is, the number of nurses on the books and those in training; of these, she would report the number off sick, on sick leave, on holiday and special leave. She would then bring out those items of her weekly business that needed the House Committee's approval and consent. Her administrative duties were weighty but she was a nurse at heart and did not neglect her work on the wards. Ward visiting was more than a routine; she would find the time to speak to individual patients and to advise senior nurses and guide juniors. She constantly kept herself involved, at a hospital and national level, in the development of the training courses for nurses. Life was good for Miss MacManus, and she was good for nursing, working tirelessly for the profession. She was elected to the Council of the Royal College of Nursing, the National Council of Nurses of Great Britain, and the General Nursing Council for England and Wales. She had become a highly respected figure who had great influence within the profession. She also became a member of the Voluntary Advisory Nursing Board for HM Prisons. The Board held its meetings at the Women's Prison, Holloway.

On Wednesday 12 May 1937, she attended the crowning of the Duke of York as King George VI in Westminster Abbey. As Matron of Guy's Hospital, and in the company of many other colleagues in the nursing world, she was allotted a seat in the galleries. But once again the clouds of war were looming. Early in 1939 all the matrons from the big London teaching hospitals were called to Whitehall to be instructed on the war strategy for hospitals. The Minister of Health had created the Emergency Medical Service to co-ordinate a countrywide medical initiative. For administrative purposes, London was to be divided into ten sectors. The sectors circled outer London anti-clockwise and finished at sector X, which was based at Guy's Hospital. Guy's Hospital was to be evacuated, taken over for the war effort. In each of the three large hospitals of Kent County Council, the Ministry of Health proposed to build a 'hutted' unit of five hundred beds complete with operating theatres and X-ray rooms. These units would be staffed with doctors and nurses from Guy's. The Ministry proposed to conscript staff for an entirely new nursing service to be known as the Civil Nursing Reserve, a service that worked well.

Matron MacManus was based in Orpington, where she stayed at Boundary House in the grounds of the Orpington Institution for aged folk. There she waited for the casualties to arrive, but this war was different from the First World War. To begin with there was not the bombing that had been expected; the period was described as the 'phoney' war. Huge effort had been put into increasing the bed capacities in hospitals all over the country, but there were no patients. A far-reaching strategy was in place for civil defence, against gas attack, bombing, invasion, all sorts of disasters, but nothing seemed to be happening. However, events in France were moving fast. With news of Dunkirk came a sudden realization that the men of the British Expeditionary Force were in dire peril.

On the evening of 29 May 1940, Miss MacManus was one member of a small volunteer group heading for Dover, where the worst cases from the boats were coming in. Late in the evening they started work, and Miss MacManus was once again confronted with humanity's brutal behaviour. She would not forget easily the tragic sight in the wards of desperately ill men. Their injuries were horrendous; many had their faces and hands blackened with burns from burning oil on the water. Eighteen men lost their lives in a single night.

Once Dover was under control, Miss MacManus returned to Guy's. Then came the Blitz. On 7 September, enemy bombers broke though British defences and set London alight. Miss MacManus saw fires stretched before her, raging from Woolwich to London Bridge. She thought that there could not have been such a sight since the Great Fire of 1666, but London was to see even worse. A week later Guy's itself was bombed. The wide stone stairway in the medical block and the two flanking lifts came down in a cascade of great slabs of masonry and splintered wood. The people of the borough rushed in to help, and in twenty minutes all the patients had been taken, via the fire staircases, to comparative safety. This venerable building, which played such an important role in the life of Miss MacManus, was to sustain more damage.

By now Matron MacManus was sleeping underground in the Matron's house. They had converted the basement into a ground floor flat, so it withstood many other air raids. On 29 December 1940, Guy's and the neighbouring warehouses took a heavy battering from bombs and incendiaries. A full moon lit up the area, but a low spring tide meant that the Thames water level was too low for the firemen's hoses to reach. Fire raged in an uncontrollable ring around Guy's Hospital and, for the first time since it opened in 1725, the patients had to be evacuated. The following year fire once again challenged Guy's longevity, carrying off the beautiful old east wing, the courtroom, committee rooms, and Superintendent's House, with its magnificent mahogany staircase.

Now heading towards retirement, with a lifetime of profound experiences under her belt, Matron MacManus was elected President of the Royal College of Nursing in 1942. In that office until 1944, she travelled throughout the country speaking at various functions and attending meetings. In the summer of 1943 she accepted an invitation to tour Scotland, speaking to members of the Scottish section of the Royal College, and to student nurses in Edinburgh, Glasgow, Perth and Aberdeen. Matron MacManus taught with a zest for life and with humour and humility; it was hard to imagine all that she had lived through.

Following the war, life started to return to normality. Guy's Hospital was re-built and once again stood proud in its city. Miss MacManus retired five years after her expected retirement date. It was the summer of 1946 when the warm speeches were made, the leaving gifts presented, the letters of affection written and a godspeed read. She drove out of the front of Guy's to her retirement in County Mayo in Ireland.

Reminiscing, she reflected on a day when she was doing her ward round and met an old Guy's nurse who was then a patient. When she approached the bed, she asked the woman about her memories of the old days. Matron MacManus asked her, 'Were you under Miss Victoria Jones or Miss Burt?' The old lady looked at her with piercing blue eyes. 'No, Matron, neither of those. I was under Miss Loag – and a fine matron she was!' Miss Loag was Matron at Guy's from 1852. Matron MacManus felt, as she looked down at this wonderful old lady who had really seen and worked in the legendary Guy's of those far-away days, that she was stretching out across the years – touching and greeting her predecessors. She wondered would any ancient dame say in years to come, 'I worked under Matron MacManus.'

Miss MacManus died on 22 February 1978 at the age of ninety-one. Buried in Ireland, there was a service of thanksgiving in Guy's Chapel on 10 May and a memorial service held at Southwark Cathedral on 5 June 1978. Her obituary in *The Times* of 6 March 1978 rightly described her as one of the outstanding matrons of modern times, and her cousin L.A.G. Strong described her as 'a legend, even during her term of office at Guy's'. She epitomized all that was good in traditional British nursing, and gained an OBE in 1930 and the CBE in 1947. A superb organizer, she was what might be described as quintessentially human when dealing with other people, be they her nurses, her patients, her professional colleagues or her own family.

Very family-orientated, Miss MacManus's organizational skills extended to her family as well, where she put in order both the senior and junior members of her family. Her niece, Maeve MacManus, well remembers these skills coming together at each Boxing Day. She would give a marvellous party, inviting all the family and providing her own home-made produce. These parties brought together her mother's family, the Boyds, and her father's family, the MacManuses. One tradition Emily insisted on was an after-dinner speech by the children. This was regarded by them as a dreaded ordeal! Maeve MacManus remembers being terrified when it came to her turn, but following the speech, happily, it was time for games. These would be a series of pencil and paper games that both the adults and the children could play. Later in the evening, she would play the piano and sing. Having a wide repertoire of music, Miss MacManus could entertain the whole family and would always include a rendition of

'Campdown Races'. Maeve MacManus, still singing herself at seventy, is convinced that her aunt could have been a fine mezzo-soprano had her voice not been damaged absorbing gas whilst attending the wounded during the First World War. Surgeon Rear-Admiral Forrest, a trainee medical student at Guy's Hospital in 1939, remembered her very well over sixty years later as the 'charming Irish girl'.

VI
Service Matron

Women serving in the military services is a modern concept, but women nursing the sick and injured of the military is not. William Ferguson, Inspector General of military hospitals in England in 1846, wrote that whenever it was practical, women of the army should be employed in hospitals, with their duties strictly confined to the sick wards. He explained that women may not always be found for the service of hospitals, but when they were, they ought to be employed. Attendance upon the sick and wounded was the understood condition of their being allowed to accompany the army.

Since long before even the Crimean War, the army and naval services needed, but did not always get, the best medical and nursing provision. In medieval Europe, companies of knights bound by monastic vows fought to defend Christendom. Particularly relevant to hospital nursing in the nineteenth and twentieth centuries was the Order 'of the Knights Hospitallers. The serving Brothers, and in the early days the serving Sisters, nursed the sick in hospitals. Attracting the very best of the Knights of the time and being rich, they could afford the finest for the people who needed their care. A military discipline that enforced a rigid code of conduct and demanded unquestioning obedience under-pinned all future military and civilian hospitals.

In Britain there was a contracting system between St Thomas's Hospital, St Bartholomew's Hospital and the Savoy

Hospital, London, with each hospital receiving the injured from military campaigns until the middle of the seventeenth century. As early as 1642, Parliament had opened its first dedicated military hospital at the Savoy, where there were already four sisters involved in the nursing of servicemen. The numbers were increased to fifteen female nurses with a larger number of males in supporting roles. Subsequently two further hospitals were opened, at Parsons Green in 1645 and Ely House in 1684, but the numbers for whom they could accommodate always proved inadequate. Areas outside London could not help as they were still recovering from the closure of abbeys and monasteries during the reformation. Therefore, any individual serviceman who was wounded had to rely on the goodwill of others. One such person was healer Elizabeth Alkin. She tended wounded sailors in about 1650. The sailors landed in East Anglia and she was known to have attended them at Harwich and Ipswich. A small pension was granted to her from the government, which was a notable gesture. The majority of servicemen, however, who could not find a healer, had to rely on the goodwill of local parishes, individual households or alehouses. Worse still were the 'informal' hospitals. These were large establishments of huts given over by (often unscrupulous) owners contracted to 'look after' the sick and wounded. In these places, nurses and surgeons provided minimum attention. It was to be the middle of the eighteenth century before major consideration was given to the idea of large-scale hospitals for military personnel. Male medical officers and male orderlies provided the majority of care for the sick and injured. These orderlies were generally detached from within the same regiment as the soldiers being nursed. There was an obvious benefit from this in that there was a sense of camaraderie, of looking after one's own. In some ways this was thought to make up for a lack of other skills.

By the seventeenth century, both the army and navy were employing women as nurses. Both services had travelling field hospitals to support foreign campaigns, land-based hospitals, and hospital ships. It was the practice to have female nurses on hospital ships and, in 1703, there was an order that specified that every hospital ship was to have nurses and laundresses, but none of them was to be under the age of fifty years. There was one ship, the *Syam*, which in 1703 had ten females on board, each one named.

The first usage of the title 'Matron' in military circles was associated with the hospital that was set up to care for the sick at James II's annual camp on Hounslow Heath. In 1688, the matron there received £100 per year, the sum paying for her salary and for the medicaments for sick soldiers. Although there was no military nursing service as such, there is evidence of continued employment of women for the nursing of the sick and injured of the military. By 1750 some women were making a career in army nursing. The practice of using women to nurse troops in the field was already commonplace by the turn of the eighteenth century, and in Queen Elizabeth's day women were frequently employed in military hospitals. Of where these nurses came from little is known, but what is known is that many such women were respected. Indeed, wives and widows of soldiers were highly valued as nurses by the high command of Cromwell's army. When one of the Lord Protector's leading lieutenants returned from a disastrous expedition to the West Indies, Cromwell complained, 'Had more women gone, I suppose that many [of my men] would not have perished as they did for want of care and attendance.'

The hospital ship *Lynn* was used from 1740 to 1742 at the battle of Carthegena. The ship had three separate matrons over that period, each one being in charge of up to twenty female nurse helpers who received three shillings per day. This was far more than a sergeant was paid. They were not individually named, but included on the ship's muster, a singularly notable event for women. Matron was often included on lists of general hospital staff and was sometimes noted in the army lists, suggesting that the post commanded considerable prestige. In these hospitals there was one director and one matron, with matron at the top of the nurse hierarchy. Usually the matron was based at the main hospital, overseeing a number of smaller units. In 1756 at a council held at Haslar Hospital, two matrons of the time were named, Mrs Miller and Mrs Eastwood, though little else is known about them. At the same time a Jane Brown, nurse of the middle ward, was dismissed for sleeping with four or five patients and infecting one of them with 'foul disease'. In 1758, a Dr James Lind wrote that at Haslar Hospital there were ninety women nurses and seldom less than twenty-four women constantly employed in the wash-rooms, 'all these under sober and discreet Matrons'. Indeed the instructions for the matrons of Haslar Hospital (circa 1780), written by the Commissioners for taking care of Sick and Hurt Seamen and Marines, demand that nurses be directly responsible to the matron. It was the matron's job to instruct the nurses and see that they performed their duties properly. The matron was expected to attend the wards daily to see that instructions were carried out and to check on the nurse's behaviour. Clearly matron was expected to be fully in charge.

In military establishments matron supervised the nurses, generally having more contact with individuals than any other member of staff. Donald Munro, physician to George III's army, wrote that every matron or head nurse, was to go round all the wards of the hospital at least twice a day, morning and evening. They were to see that the nurses kept their wards clean and that they behaved themselves soberly; to give due attention to their patients, and to examine the diet of their patients and see that it was well presented. If she found anything amiss, she was to report the same to the physician, surgeon or apothecary of the hospital.

The Royal Naval Medical Service magazine published a paper in 1948 giving an insight into conditions in country and military hospitals, the original paper having been written in 1789 by John Verdin. It described how military hospitals in the late eighteenth century were very much comparable to country hospitals. They could be quieter and cleaner, and where it was common for the floors to be sanded and dry-rubbed in country hospitals, the practice was avoided in military hospitals. The patients would have had white linen shirts, hospital clothing and white bed-linen. Numbers of patients in bed would have been around fifteen to eighteen hundred, but there would have been fewer per ward, perhaps only twenty. It was common practice in country hospitals to nail windows open in summer. 'All the nurses would be women, which was thought very proper, as they were cleanly and tender.' Visitors were admitted on only two days in the week. Similar to country hospitals however, 'the *inside sewers* are offensive: there are *no cisterns* in the wards'. The pipes from which they were supplied with water, both for drinking and washing, adjoined the sewers.

After 1838 women were not supposed to attend to male patients, and certainly not the middle section of the body, but in general this was disregarded. In 1854 three female applicants for service nursing posts claimed to have previous military nursing experience. One was said to have understanding and experience of gunshot wounds, another was said to have been used to nursing soldiers at Spike Island, another had been employed by the army for five years but mostly in the women's ward. Certainly in 1856 there were women nursing at the Woolwich Arsenal Hospital.

Throughout the nineteenth century, more and more army bungling led to the deterioration of already inadequate resources in hospital services. Not having learned lessons from earlier campaigns, particularly the eighteenth century Spanish and Dutch conflicts, experienced male nursing staff were still being called away to fight, leaving inexperienced and often seriously debilitated soldiers as replacements.

The Army Nursing Service came into being in 1881. The headquarters were to be the Royal Victoria Hospital, Netley, built at the time of the Crimean War. This was a hospital that Miss Nightingale did not like because she felt it faced the wrong way (north-east), and that it was poorly ventilated. She was proved right. However the hospital must have held some fondness for those who worked there, as it became affectionately known as the 'cradle' of the Army Nursing Service.

Mrs Jane C. Deeble entered Netley Hospital in 1869 along with six other Nightingale nurses. She was the widow of an officer who was killed in Abyssinia. In 1880 she was appointed Superintendent. It was to be her role to introduce training for a number of nurses at Netley; these were to be nursing sisters trained in military nursing. The type of women that Mrs Deeble wanted were those who would be 'terrors to any wrongdoer'. Rebecca Strong was an outstanding nurse from St Thomas's Hospital. She had been among a group of nurses sent to the Royal Hospital, Netley, under Mrs Deeble in 1869. A natural success there, she was then appointed Matron of the Royal Hospital, Glasgow. In 1879 Mrs Deeble took sixteen nurses to the Zulu War in South Africa; they took over the newly built hospital at Addigton. In all, Mrs Deeble remained at Netley for twenty years. She was later famous for leading a party of twenty-four nurses to Egypt to assist the British forces under Lord Wolseley. She found that conditions for the sick and wounded soldiers had not improved much, and set about a successful programme of improvement. A committee of inquiry was set up to examine the problem, and Miss Nightingale again provided essential advice. Later Mrs Deeble was appointed Superintendent of the Army Nursing Service. Miss Norman took her place at Netley.

Belle Storey was head nurse for the navy at Haslar Hospital, Gosport. Miss Storey proved to be such a success that a rose was named after her in 1984, to mark the centenary of the Naval Nursing Service. (Many naval nursing staff proudly display the rose in their gardens.) Haslar Hospital, Gosport, was the headquarters of the Naval Nursing Sisters, with Miss Louisa Hogg superintending. Miss Whistler, a sister of the well-known artist, was Superintendent of Plymouth and Chatham naval hospitals in the 1880s. By 1888, Lady Superintendents were taking groups of nurses to places such as Rawalpindi and Bangalore, Meerut and Lucknow. In particular, Miss Lock became Senior Lady Superintendent for military services in India.

Until the Crimean War, there had been no awards given to women in nursing. Throughout history, many women had lost their lives in selfless devotion to the injured and sick. Queen Victoria, however, rectified this. The Royal Red Cross was an order instituted by Queen Victoria, on St George's Day in 1883, for the purpose of rewarding nurses who gave special service. The award, to this day, is conferred 'upon any lady, whether subject or foreign person, who may be recommended by Our Secretary of State for War for special exertions in providing for the nursing of sick and wounded soldiers and sailors of Our Army and Navy'. The clause 'or Our Air Force' was added later. The decoration consists of a red Maltese cross bearing the words Faith, Hope and Charity. Some of the early recipients of the Red Cross were Florence Nightingale, Mrs Deeble and Miss H. Campbell Norman.

There were two nursing groups ready to meet the needs of the expected conflict of the First World War: Queen Alexandra's Imperial Military Nursing Service (Dame Ethel Hope Beecher was Matron-in-Chief, and was in close contact with the British War Office); and Queen Alexandra's Royal Naval Nursing Service (QARNNS), who supplied the naval nursing care needs. Princess Mary's Royal Air Force Nursing Service (PMRAFNS) did not come into existence until 1918.

Miss Joan Woodgate was born on 30 August 1912. Her father was Sir Alfred Woodgate CBE, and her mother was called Louise Alice. Miss Woodgate was educated at Surbiton High School, Surrey, and was the youngest of a large family. As Miss Woodgate was doing very well at school, her headmistress tried to talk her into a career as a schoolteacher. Digging in her heels, and having seen her half-sister in her nurse's uniform (she was a nurse at King's College Hospital, London), she was determined to pursue her own ambition of becoming a nurse.

Miss Woodgate trained for four years at St George's Hospital, London, from 1932 onwards. She had previously attended an interview at Guy's Hospital with Matron Emily MacManus. Miss Woodgate described Miss MacManus as a most handsome woman who looked very kind and caring. Greeted by a warm smile, Matron MacManus listened to her most intently. Miss Woodgate was only eighteen years old and rather slim. At the end of the interview she was told by Miss MacManus that she would have to take an untrained nursing post for one year; this was to see if she could withstand the physical demands of nursing, because Miss MacManus felt that she looked too frail to be able to undertake the hardships of nurse training. Many years later when Miss Woodgate was Superintendent Sister at Plymouth, a young naval cadet came to the hospital and stated that he had a famous aunt who had been the matron of Guy's Hospital. He was obviously very proud of her and stated that she was none other than Emily MacManus. Miss Woodgate said to him, 'Next time you see your aunt tell her that you have met Miss Woodgate, whom she turned down many years before for being too frail for nursing. Tell her she is now in the Queen's Naval Nursing Service, and has never had a day off sick in her life.'

Determined to become a nurse, Miss Woodgate commenced training at St George's, Hyde Park Corner, where Miss Hanks was Matron. She remembers Miss Hanks always having two Pekinese dogs with her. Living in the nurses' home in the 1930s was enjoyable and had a good community life. The trainees worked from seven in the morning until a quarter to nine at night, with two hours off. 'It seems hard now to the modern girl but it was the custom of the time.' They were treated strictly but then Miss Woodgate had been treated strictly at home. They enjoyed their off-duty time and spent most of their money (£20 per annum) on food. Hyde Park was nearby and there were usually complimentary tickets for the theatre, but they would have had to be back by ten.

It was compulsory for the staff to rise at ten minutes to six with breakfast at half-past six. All staff were registered in the dining room. Chapel was at ten to seven, and from there they went straight on to their wards. From the very beginning they were told quite clearly by Matron Hanks that the most important person in the hospital was the patient, and Miss Woodgate pointed out that in those days, nurses *wanted* to nurse the patients, they were there *for* the patients. They served all the meals so they knew exactly what had been eaten and who was not eating. 'It will be hard for the modern girl to understand but we were still very innocent of the world when we began training; an eighteen-year-old may not understand that now.'

Following a year as staff nurse and then an appointment as Ward Sister at Queen Charlotte's Hospital, Miss Woodgate joined QARNNS as a nursing sister in 1938. She was twenty-five. Her intention was to travel, and she did. 'I was lucky and served a lot of my time overseas in the Middle East and Far East.' When Miss Woodgate first started in Plymouth, the sailors did not have sick leave; they had to stay in hospital until they were fit for duty. As they were not very well staffed in those days, if they had a good galley hand for example, he was 'worth his weight in gold'. They would find some way to hang on to him. 'You would say to the medical staff, "please don't send old ... home yet, he is too valuable to us." So with luck we would have him until a replacement took over.'

Miss Woodgate served in Alexandria at the 64th General Hospital from 1941 until 1944. The main hospital had been previously a boys' public school and remains so once again. The main part was hutted, with six hundred army beds under the authority of an army matron, and six hundred naval beds under the charge of Miss Woodgate. The army matron was much older than Miss Woodgate, and very experienced, proving extremely helpful to her. Miss Woodgate had over twenty nursing sisters and twenty VADs. Being so many miles from any support they just had to get on with their work, there was no one to check whether they were doing the right thing or not. Fortunately, Miss Woodgate found that the ward sisters were very good.

The most worrying time for her was when Rommel was breaking through towards Alexandria and they had to start making evacuation plans. The Fleet Medical Officer immediately sent for her. Along with two naval medical officers, they were told to prepare a list of half of their staff who could be evacuated in four hours' time. It proved to be not quite the problem that it seemed at first. Not too experienced, she relied on the experience of the army matron who proved to be very helpful. The army matron and Miss Woodgate decided to make a cup of tea and retire to their respective sitting-rooms to go through their lists. Miss Woodgate put all the VADs on the list because they had been away since 1939 and so were due to return home, and also some of the sisters, but everyone came to her and said they were not going. In the end they did not have to implement their plan.

Near the fighting they would still often receive wounded men in fairly good condition. This was because they had already been through the advanced dressing station. The men would have a label on them stating their injury and treatment; those with tourniquets would have a red cross on their forehead, a signal that they required immediate attention. There were many deaths at Alexandria, and on the death of a patient Miss Woodgate would write to the next of kin, often receiving touching letters in return. She felt this gratitude was due partly to mothers, sweethearts and wives knowing that their boys had not died in a ditch or on the sand. What she also thought very important was that, in a hospital, the men had women looking after them. One New Zealand family corresponded with her after their son had died and asked if she had a mother in England, and if so, where did she live. When she wrote back they sent a parcel of food to her mother and continued doing so regularly until the end of the war.

In the hospital they had a mixed group of patients, both allies and prisoners, and Miss Woodgate found the Australians to be 'a wonderful bunch of men' but not very amenable to discipline. They would walk around with nothing on their top half and it used to infuriate the army matron. She remembered having an inspection of their huts. When they got to the huts, the Medical Officer said to the Inspection Officer, 'I do not know what we will find when we go in here, they are all Australians!' The sister had said to these men that if they let her down, she would kill them. The inspectors went in and it was as if the men were on guard parade. They had cleared everything. Those who were in bed sat to attention, and those standing by their beds stood to attention. The inspectors never knew what to expect.

Miss Woodgate was then shore-based at the Royal Naval College, and then at HMS *Westcliff* until 1945 when she joined HMHS *Empire Clyde* for two years, sailing from Scotland with a party of Australian ex-POWs and a unit of

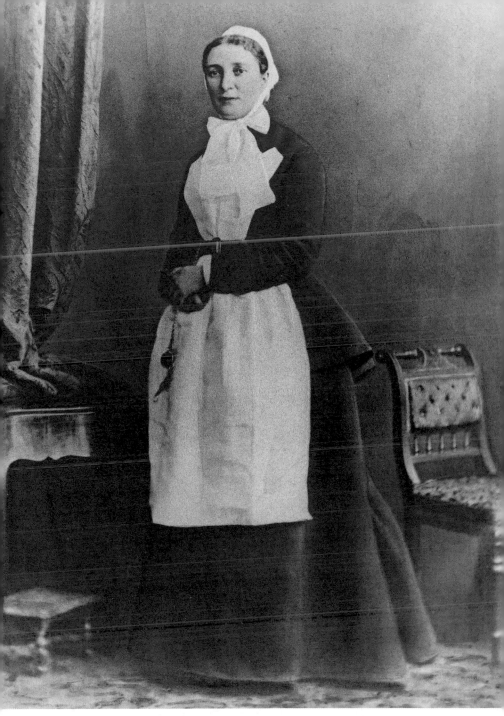

Sister Dora, the outstanding nurse of Walsall in the 1870s. Note the 'Sister Dora Cap' worn by generations of nurses

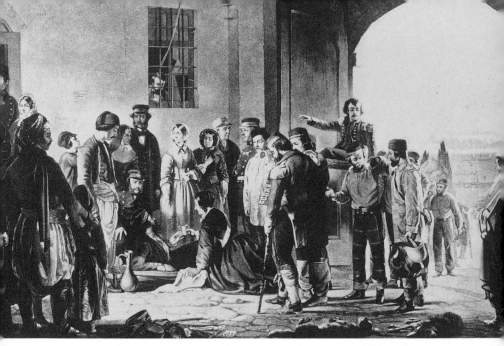

Florence Nightingale at Scutari depicted in a painting entitled 'The ministering angel of the Crimean War' by Jerry Barratt and Samuel Bellini

Miss H. Campbell Norman, lady superintendent of the army nursing staff, 1897. She wears the Egypt medal with clasp and also the Royal Red Cross

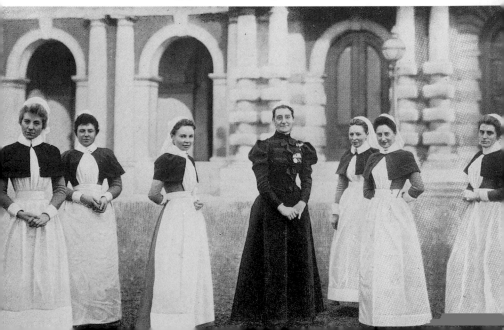

Mary Cadbury, matron of Queen's Hospital, Birmingham, *c.* 1890

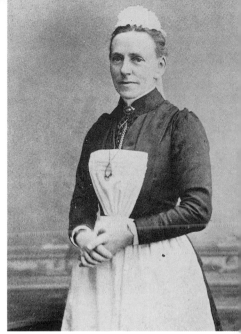

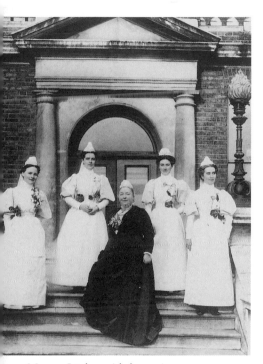

Matron Lückes with her assistants at The London Hospital. On her right is Miss Monks, appointed matron following Miss Lückes' death in 1919. On her extreme left is Miss Littleboy appointed matron in 1931 following the retirement of Miss Monks

Ethel Gordon Manson (later Mrs Bedford Fenwick), matron at St Bartholomew's Hospital, 1881–7

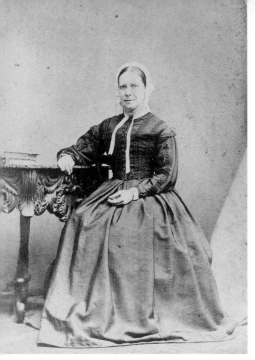

Agnes Jones, nurse superintendent of Brownlow Infirmary, Liverpool, 1866–9. One of the first nurse martyrs

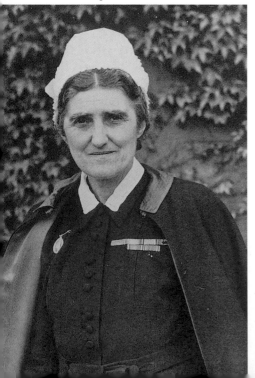

Emily MacManus, matron of Guy's Hospital, 1927–46

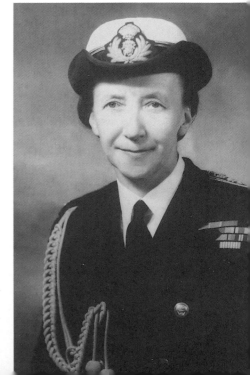

Joan Woodgate, matron-in-chief of the QARNNS, 1962–6

Matron Julia Massey with the Duchess of York in the presence of Surgeon Rear-Admiral D.A. Lammiman LVO and Surgeon Rear-Admiral F. Golden OBE, 1989

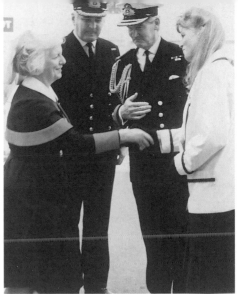

Mary Butland in her prized armoured corps black beret, 1942

Matron Mary Butland at her retirement from nursing in 1963

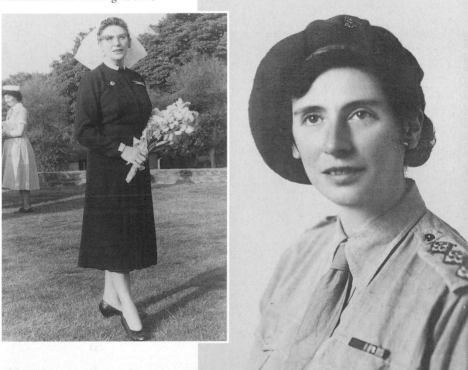

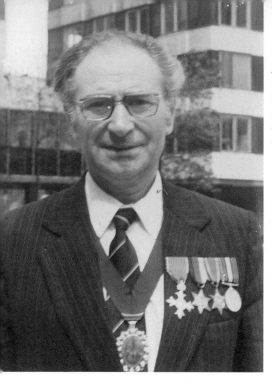

John Greene OBE, wearing the 1939–45 war service medal the Burma Star, and the ribbon and badge as president of the Association of Nurse Administrators (formerly the Matrons' Association)

Left to right: Argentinian medical officer; Captain Geoff Clark, SS *Uganda*; Miss Edith Meiklejohn, matron, QARNNS; Andrew Rintoul, Royal Navy medical officer-in-charge

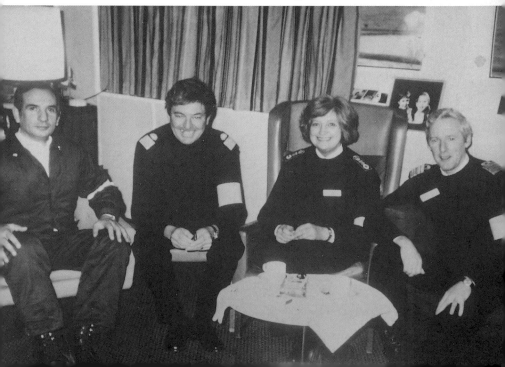

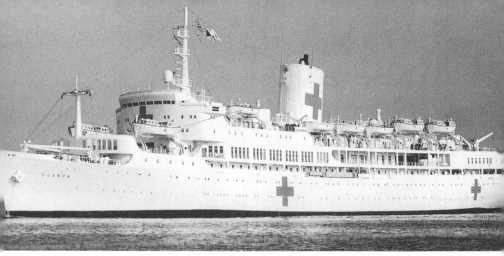

SS *Uganda* destined for the Falkland Islands following refit to the hospital ship

Commander Gillian Comrie, 1996, matron of RFA *Argus* in the Gulf War, 1991

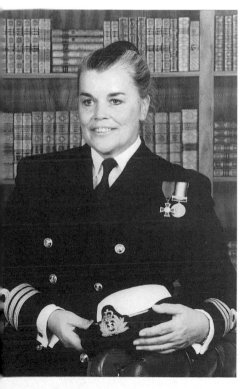

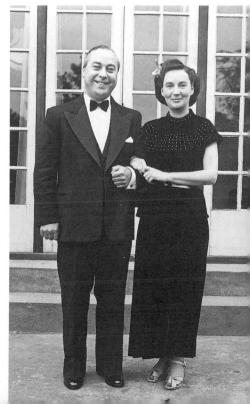

Lionel and Beryl Lewis in 1943, master and matron of St James's Hospital, Gravesend, shortly after escaping a major enemy bomb incident

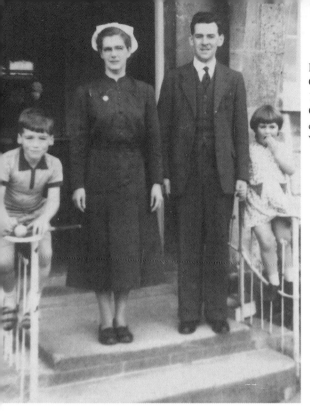

Betty Connor, matron, and Bill Connor, superintendent, in 1959 with their children Geoffrey and Joan on the steps of their home at Stow-on-the-Wold

Monica Matterson (*second from left*) and Ann Escolme, matron (*centre*) at nurses' prize-giving, Scarborough Hospital, 1947.

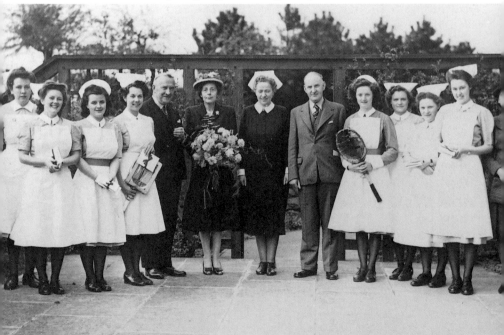

New Zealand sisters, taking them home. She then joined the British Pacific Fleet just as the war ended, spending time in Hong Kong before returning to Malta where the ship was re-commissioned in 1947. After two years in England, she sailed east towards Korea on HMHS *Maine* from 1952-54. The Korean War (1950-53) ended soon after their arrival in Japan. This was followed by a further six postings between England, Hong Kong and Malta in shore-based hospitals and hospital ships. As matron on a hospital ship, she had to have good social skills because the nurses could not get out of each other's way. Matron's role was also different in shore-based hospitals because they lived with the sisters and dined in the same mess. She always had great respect for the sisters and nurses because at this time the navy and naval medicine were still very much male domains. She always felt lucky to have been in QARNNS.

Following appointments as Principal Matron at RNH (Royal Navy Hospital) Haslar and RNH Malta, Miss Woodgate was then appointed Matron-in-Chief of QARNNS in 1962, staying in the post until her retirement in 1966. It was mainly an office job. State-enrolled nurse training commenced during her time in that post. As Matron-in-Chief Miss Woodgate missed hospital life terribly. It was very much an administrative job dealing mainly with staff records. It always amazed her that reports were so uniform, although she found the men invariably (and not surprisingly) over-marked women, but the other two matrons-in-chief (army and air force) could also see through this. The seriousness of those reports always worried her, how someone could damn another person professionally with only the stroke of a pen.

One surprise for Miss Woodgate when she was appointed Matron-in-Chief was that she had to start cleaning her own shoes and making her own bed. Throughout her nursing and serving life in the navy, she had always been used to maids. 'Then suddenly I had to do everything. One time I flew back from the north and had to take the dustbin out at the back of the street when I got back. I thought, well this must be very good for you!'

Miss Woodgate was awarded the RRC, CBE and Order of St John. (Queen Victoria, under a Royal Charter of 1888, incorporated the Order of St John of Jerusalem to the United Kingdom. The insignia is awarded for voluntary work in connection with the Priory's activities in hospital, ambulance and relief work.) On her retirement, Miss Woodgate was appointed to the War Graves Commission from 1966 until 1983. It was an appointment made by the Queen, and Miss Woodgate was the first female to be given this opportunity. It proved to be a very interesting and rewarding time for her. The work of the commission not only involves maintaining war graves, but also organizing the burials of recently located bodies of servicemen, and, using their extensive records, names for people searching for graves of relatives.

Having travelled so much already it was a while before Miss Woodgate started doing that again. She concentrated mainly on her gardening and country pursuits before returning to Alexandria and other places she had visited as a QARNNS.

In the military services the post of 'matron' continued well beyond those of other hospitals, and Julia Massey, originally trained as a nurse at the University College Hospital, London, was one of the last to have this post at RNH Haslar, Gosport. She had a service background: her father had been in the Royal Naval Air Service in the First World War, and her brother Timothy had served in the Merchant Navy and was a submariner in the Royal Navy Reserve. Julia joined QARNNS in July 1968.

Following a varied career in RN hospitals and establishments throughout England and abroad, Miss Massey RRC was promoted to Chief Nursing Officer, and appointed Matron of RNH Haslar. Following promotion to Principal Nursing Officer, she spent five years in the Headquarters of the Medical Director General (Naval). When QARNNS rank titles changed, she held the rank of Captain. As matron of RNH Haslar, Miss Massey was responsible for providing the highest standard of nursing care to service personnel, both serving and retired, and civilians within the Gosport area. To achieve this aim, she had an 'open door' policy for the nursing officers and staff nurses in the wards and departments. She believed in the importance of her being available for her staff, and able to sort out issues there and then. Knowing her staff individually was very important in achieving this end. Like any other matron she met regularly with the staff to discuss issues, develop protocol, and ensure that their nursing standards and equipment were of the highest quality, and that they remained up-to-date. At this time matrons were also beginning to have a financial responsibility for their role.

As RNH Haslar provided training experience for student nurses and the probationary royal naval medical assistants, it was important to ensure that the hospital provided the best experience and support possible. Being the senior officer within the hospital, Miss Massey had overall responsibility for QARNNS ratings; this task was discharged through the royal naval division system. Nursing officers were responsible for the nurses' general welfare. In particular they wrote reports on their progress and made certain that they undertook training both professional and for the services, leading to advancement within their service. Miss Massey in turn wrote reports on the nursing officers and, working together with the medical officer-in-charge (MOIC), these reports were used to select officers for further commissions and promotion. Each week, together with the MOIC and other personnel, Massey undertook 'rounds', visiting about five different areas of the hospital. Not only did this involve the clinical areas, but also accommodation and recreation areas, the galley, stores and cellars. It took six months to cover the whole hospital, examining the fabric of the place, meeting staff, and listening to problems.

Following retirement, Miss Massey became Chairman of QARNNS Officers' Association and now shares responsibility for QARNNS archives at the Institute of Naval Medicine.

I left the hospital on promotion to Captain, and remained in QARNNS a further six years. My appointment as Matron of

Haslar Hospital I regard as the pinnacle of my career, and can only describe leaving the clinical environment, and sitting behind a desk, as akin to a bereavement.

VII

A Moment in History

To find a human example of the bravery shown by people in the nursing profession, and of the courageous response of women (in particular) in times of national crisis, we need look no further than the following lady, Miss Jane Butland. The following story comes very much from Miss Butland's own words, as well as the personal diaries she kept.

Miss Catherine Mary Butland RRC, known to her friends as Jane, was born in Torquay in 1903. She was the youngest of four sisters, all benefiting from their father's liberal attitudes. He made it clear that they should all do something useful with their lives, so the girls were educated accordingly. Miss Butland and one of her sisters chose nursing as a career, the other two chose teaching. Her father, the late C. Butland, was a captain in the army, and well-known in Coventry for his work as conductor of the City of Coventry Police Band. Her mother was from a naval background and was greatly involved in charitable work. The Butlands are an old family and can be traced back as far as 1115. Living on the moors at Holme, near Ashburton, people did not move around much in the early centuries. It was not until the middle of the seventeenth century that people began to move into the area. The first of the family to leave the area were her grandfather's parents who moved to Torquay.

Miss Butland spent her infancy in India but was educated privately in Torquay until the age of eleven. She then went on to grammar school where she studied until she was sixteen.

'Back in the twenties there was little for a girl to do. I spent two years in a commercial college doing shorthand, typing, bookkeeping and commercial French, and then spent two weeks in an office. It was enough to convince me that I did not want to do that as a career.' Miss Butland started her nursing career aged eighteen, in a small children's hospital in Rodney Street, Liverpool. She started her formal nurse training at St Bartholomew's Hospital, London, in 1923, under the controversial Matron Miss Annie Mackintosh, who was appointed in 1910. Miss Mackintosh began her career as matron with a slight disadvantage: she followed the great Isla Stewart, who had trained at the Nightingale School of Nursing and was a friend of Miss Nightingale. Controversy also surrounded her because she had only completed two years of nurse training. On her retirement in 1927, however, she had proven herself to be more than capable for the job. This was a world still steeped in unfaltering respect for one's superiors. It was also a world of uncontested discipline. Miss Mackintosh would always notify the wards that she was on her way and was always escorted by someone, usually her assistant matron. Miss Butland pointed out that if a nurse was sent on an errand, for example to the dispensary, and she met matron half-way, she would stop and say, 'May I escort you to where you are going, Matron?' and she did; it was seen as old-world courtesy.

To train at St Bartholomew's Hospital, Miss Butland had to be supported by her family. This was at a time when a girl felt lucky to be accepted for training, and it was deemed a privilege to be able to nurse. It had become an elite occupation for proud women in a world where they could be more equal. Her salary was five pounds a year. Although the material was provided for the uniform, it still had to be made to the hospital's instruction and cost one shilling. The dresses had to be ten inches off the ground with a seven-inch hem and three one-inch tucks; these were carefully measured before the dresses could be worn.

Having experienced a happy and healthy childhood, Miss Butland was suddenly exposed to all manner of infections. 'I was never well the whole time. I don't know how they ever let me finish. But we were always well looked after when we trained. It was a twelve-hour day with two hours off in the morning or afternoon. We also had to be able to cook because the nurses and the maid cooked all the vegetables on the ward.' Miss Butland feels that as nurses they were taught cleanliness thoroughly. It was probably the most important aspect of training. 'I was recently ill myself and in hospital; for five days a dirty tissue lay under a dusty bed. The cleaner was not under the control of the ward sister but the domestic supervisor, and the domestic supervisor was not based at the hospital. What nonsense!'

At St Bartholomew's ward sisters still had their bedrooms attached to the ward; they never left. The night nurse had to clean the bath every night because the ward sister would use it. Sister would walk through the ward in her dressing-gown and would expect to be escorted by a junior nurse. Before her bath she would count the dirty linen. It depended if the nurse liked the sister or not as to whether they put fouls in there. She would then want to be escorted back again, so the nurse had to keep a sharp look out for when she was ready. Another job for a junior nurse was to walk matron's dog. It had to be taken out at midnight for one reason, and at four in the morning for another. It did not matter *what* was happening – this job *had* to be done.

Following her training Miss Butland went, as Sister, to a cottage hospital in Welling. This was a small hospital in comparison to St Bartholomew's, and for this reason it proved to be a vastly different experience for her. The rigorous routine that had been more familiar to her was now replaced by a slightly more casual approach where the matron undertook a wide range of 'medical' tasks. Matron's rooms were just inside the main door. In one room, normally her sitting-room, she would deal with all the casualties; there was no one else to do it; there was no resident doctor. They had one doctor on call, but he might be out on his rounds, so matron had to be able to put her hand to anything, and she did.

Later, when Miss Butland was Sister at another hospital, she found herself back in the strict codes of moral conduct dating from the Nightingale years. One day she had a late pass to go and see her sister in Coventry. To make the party numbers up she invited a doctor along. The day the pass was to be used, Matron sent for her. She said, 'Is it true that you are taking a doctor with you?' to which Miss Butland replied, 'Yes, that is correct.' Matron said, 'Well, I am sorry, I am going to revoke your late pass. Butland asked why, and Matron replied, 'If there were an accident, think of it, you and a medical officer.' So, 'in a fit of temper', Miss Butland said, 'Obviously you do not trust me to run the ward either, so please accept my resignation.' And she did resign. 'If I was responsible as a ward sister, and I was, I felt I was also responsible as a person.'

At the outbreak of the Second World War, Miss Butland, now Assistant Matron, joined the Territorial Army and was sent to mobilize a casualty clearing station in Torquay. Here she found growing tension, excitement and fear for the future, and also considered the overt lunacy of war. She was a nurse, a care provider, but was having to prepare for the reception of anticipated war casualties. Before Miss Butland was allowed to embark on the ship to her first posting, she was given a survival talk in the event of the ship sinking. After impressing on the men and women the rule that their iron ration (tinned food) could only be opened in an emergency and only on the orders of an officer, the instructor then continued, 'but if we are torpedoed, and you are in the water for more than twenty-four hours, you may open your rations without waiting for an officer's orders.' She had visions of the poor soldiers swimming around the Channel clutching a tin of rations in one hand and a penny, which was needed to open the tin, in the other. 'But we dare not laugh!'

Miss Butland was in Belgium working as a theatre sister in a field hospital when Germany invaded. The hospital unit was given just half an hour to evacuate and then a German officer blew up the bridge that was to be their escape route. After the evacuation, for two weeks the field hospital was isolated from the allies. The unit remained in Belgium until its harrowing evacuation from Dunkirk. The unit had its injured with it, but it was greatly hampered on the journey by the civilian population. They were all over the roads, walking with bundles or pushing carts. The unit frequently had to stop and take cover from bombing and machine-gunning. Fortunately it suffered no casualties, but the same could not be said of the refugees. At Dunkirk itself and along the beaches it was practically non-stop bombing during daylight hours; in the nurses' opinion, the ambulance train seemed a definite object of attack. The team left on the very last hospital ship, war-torn and drained, both relieved and stressed by the experience. Those days in Belgium were the hardest Miss Butland spent in her whole life; it was absolute pressure the whole time. There was so little they could do with so many injured, just clean up the entrance and exit holes of the wounds and pack them with sulphonamide; that was it, that was all they could do. It was almost like a production line and the nurses could not allow themselves to become too emotional. Many nurses were left with psychiatric problems resulting from this horrific experience.

On 14 November 1940, Miss Butland went on leave. The RAF flew her from Ireland to an airfield on the outskirts of Coventry where her parents were then living. She landed at about four in the afternoon on that fateful day. She quickly ascertained that her parents were staying with her married sister, out in the country. Her brother collected her on the way to his house. That night was very noisy with gunfire and bombing. Very early in the morning, Miss Butland and her brother-in-law set off for the city to see what damage had been done, particularly to the house. 'I can honestly say that nothing I had seen in France compared to the damage and destruction that I found when we arrived on that morning.' In one night the lives of 520 men, women and children were lost and more than 1,200 people were seriously injured. Matron Joyce Burton and Sister Emma Horne of the Coventry General Hospital both received the George Medal for disregarding their own safety that night, continuing to perform their duties under the most extreme dangers.

After the short break in England, undeterred by her experience in Belgium, Miss Butland was posted to the Middle East. Now Captain in the QUAIMNS she was to head one of the first mobile hospitals used in wartime. No.1 Mobile Military Unit, named the 'Freak Unit'. Her diary notes:

> No. 1 Mobile was a great headache to Headquarters. The British Army had never had anything like it before. We were neither a Casualty Clearing Station, nor a Base Hospital. We had no pre-determined level of staffing, and being American equipped, we had no standard equipment. I am sure it must have been a joy to the Quartermaster, since we did not have to account for any losses.

This fully equipped, pre-packed component of one hundred beds was intended as a 'long-duration' field hospital. The unit could be expanded by erecting tents as required and nursing patients on stretchers instead of in beds. An average of three hundred and fifty beds were available, but at one time there were as many as eight hundred occupied beds. The basic package needed four lorries, each containing twenty-five beds and rations. Accompanying them were seven doctors of consultant rank, and two despatch riders. This was the brain-child of Montgomery. He believed that one should take the doctors and nurses to the patient, not the other way around.[1]

The field hospital was often positioned hundreds of miles from the base hospital. For this reason they could rarely evacuate back to base; instead casualties had to be moved with them. When a battle was expected, the Medical Commanding Officer would send one of the despatch riders to assess the situation at the front. From this reconnaissance, they could work out what hospital support was needed and despatch components accordingly. They could then send one or two trucks of twenty-five beds, complete with nurses and all the equipment and rations needed for three days. When camped, the tents had to be spaced a quarter of a mile apart because the Germans used to drop flares, which the nurses called 'Flaming Onions'. They could cope with one tent fire but not several at once, and with the constant scarcity of resources they could hardly risk losing any more. Because of not being able to use lights in the tents, the nurses had to start the day early and end the day early; they normally started work at five in the morning. They constantly had to deal with a terrible shortage of water; the same bowl of water would have to go round twenty-five beds. At one point, all they had was half a pint of water a day to clean with. The kitchen used the other half-pint. The nurses had to use this water for everything; teeth-cleaning, washing, and they even had to keep what they had used so they could 'wash' their clothes at the end of the week. As can be imagined, the first thing they wanted when they stopped was a shower. There was a Heath Robinson type contraption rigged up that was next to useless, but fortunately they had a Major who had somehow acquired a pig trough, so the nurses used to get invited for tea, and a bathe in the pig trough.

The 7th Army Nursing Sisters of No.1 Mobile Military Hospital were the only British women to have made a desert crossing as part of the 8th Army. They had already covered a staggering 1,221 miles since leaving Alexandria seven weeks previously. Not only that, Miss Butland and her nurses had further pushed the boundaries of what women could do and they were not fully aware at the time of the effect their presence was having on the men in the desert, but the impact was very apparent in the following tribute. The most moving experience the nurses had came after a big tank battle at Naras. The hospital team was on the move forward and they pulled in to make a meal amidst a group of tank men resting after the battle. The soldiers were so surprised to see the field hospital and the nurses ('Blimey, female nurses!') that when the tanks moved out they arranged them in single file, every tank dipping its guns in salute. It was a most moving experience and caused many tears amongst the nurses, these men who had been through so much showing such respect to the nurses. This was undoubtedly an act of comradeship from the fighting men and not an act of chivalry.

Miss Butland and the sisters were taught the use of a pistol and, as she was in charge, Miss Butland was the only one to be permanently issued with one. The issue of a gun was essentially for self-defence of both herself and her staff, but also was symbolic of the growing confidence in women, that they could now be trusted with guns, although her diary notes:

> About two in the morning I heard stealthy footsteps outside my bedroom. I called out to know who it was and was asked in return who I was. I replied, 'British Nurse.' The answer came, 'That's a good one!' I again asked but there was no reply, the footsteps came closer. I warned I would shoot but it made no difference, so I shot a round into a nearby sandbag. Great consternation ensued with the guard [turning up]. It transpired that an Officer and Sergeant were looking for a lost dog. I kept my pistol!

Often having to sleep in the ambulances when on the move, nights could be cold. Huddled in several blankets and clutching hot water bottles, they were able to remain fairly warm. On their way to Tripoli they had a special moment. The dog, Bessie, who had been with them on their desert journey, decided it was time to give birth. They could not stop, so she had to manage as well as she could in a wooden box at Miss Butland's feet. Miss Butland noted, 'Bessie surely made history in the dog world by producing nine puppies while we made our night move to Tripoli.'

After two years in the desert they were all ready for a rest; both the staff and vehicles were showing enormous strain and required timely maintenance, but after only a short break they were off again. Whilst in Tripoli they heard that the staff of No. 1 MMH were to be granted the privilege of wearing the Black Beret of No. 7 Armoured Division by special authority of General Montgomery, in recognition of their achievement and commitment. These were taken from them some months later when War Office protocol objected, but Miss Butland kept hers.

They moved far into the desert to Ben Gardane where she noted,

Ben Gardane village was beyond description, filthy. Its flies were both larger and more numerous than any we had seen since leaving Egypt. We established our hospital of between 300 and 400 beds. Here we remained during the fighting in the Mareth Line. We were now taking patients of all nationalities, both allied and enemy. All were nursed in the same tents. No special precautions were taken over enemy patients. Unfortunately the German propaganda machine had been filling the young soldiers' heads with 'never surrender' material.

The German prisoners were full of wild ideas about the treatment allegedly meted out to them. One group had been told, and believed, that the nurses had wired the mouths of all prisoners in order to prevent them from talking. The allied tactical offensive continued, and during the last days of March and the first four days of April, Miss Butland recorded that:

We admitted 1,032 patients. The whole of this time our bombers were continuously passing overhead, laying their 'carpet' and returning for more bombs. On 7 April the unit had the heaviest day in its history. This was during the Mareth Battle. On this day 1,269 patients passed through the unit. We dealt with just over 3,000 during the week. The theatre worked non-stop for four days. All transport on the way back to Tripoli was stopped by the Military Police to take the injured from us. However, with ceaseless dedication and stoic determination of the nurses, every single man was fed, even those being evacuated. The surface sand and dirt was washed off those who needed wounds dressed, and off those going to theatre.

Following months in the desert, they were delighted to reach Sousse and spend a month there. While they were at Sousse, hostilities ceased in the African campaign. Proud to have been a part of it, Miss Butland now found that it was both a thrill and a relief that the campaign had ended. The peace and quiet of that first night were uncanny. Prior to the cessation of hostilities she had taken General Miles of the

Black Cat London Division to army headquarters to say goodbye, because he was being evacuated to the UK. Miss Butland had her own staff car at that time – she was the only matron to have her own car – so she took him. She was having tea at the main army headquarters when General Von Arham sent to enquire about British terms for surrender. The reply was 'Unconditional.' 'I was told I could now go back and tell my nurses and patients. My moment in history!'

They returned via Tobruk, Amyria then to Mena and finally to Cairo. They had now travelled a total of 3,472 miles. The unit had spent 187 days on the move during its two years in the desert. In 543 days they had treated over 21,000 casualties, and there had been very few deaths. They felt that they had proved General Montgomery's philosophy right by taking the specialists to the wounded men and not the other way round.

For Miss Butland, the war was not over yet. General Montgomery was to lead the invasion against Italy. A delay in implementing operation 'Baytown' infuriated General Eisenhower, but Montgomery wanted everything in readiness, not least at No.1 Field Hospital. In the autumn of 1943, Miss Butland found herself and the field hospital moving north in support of the British Army once again. When she arrived at Alexandria she discovered that she was to head a 'special' diplomatic initiative sponsored by the Prime Minister, Winston Churchill. The unit took over a local hospital and two schools to provide accommodation for 1,000 patients from the National Liberation Army of Yugoslavia. Due to the appalling conditions in Yugoslavia, all of the patients had to be decontaminated, and their wounds were by far the worst Miss Butland had seen in the war. Her diary extracts note:

> Life could be full of surprises nursing the Yugoslavs, not least of all because of the local staff. On one occasion I was doing a ward round when I found a girl (trainee nurse) with four hand grenades fastened to her overall; another had a revolver from which she would not be parted. She had been given it as a reward for killing five German soldiers.

Later,

I am on another ward round and I get a real shock. I saw what appeared to be a gypsy encampment outside one of the tents. Small children were squatting on the ground, a baby was being fed, washing was hanging on the tent rope, and cooking utensils were spread about; a group of very excited patients were nearby. I learned from the Sister of the ward that this was the wife and family of one of the patients admitted on the previous day. The wife learned of her husband's admission and had collected together her possessions and travelled with her children many miles across the Adriatic from Yugoslavia to be near him. She was now with her husband and he would provide for her!

During the first weeks, and before her nursing numbers were increased, the staff had no time off duty, with one sister being responsible for one hundred and fifty patients. None of these patients was ambulant; they all had fractures or amputations. Most of them had been without proper nursing attention for some time and their general condition was appalling, yet the men always seemed happy and smiling. The sisters managed to find time to try and learn the odd word or two, although Tito, who was then leader of the partisans, had insisted specifically that only English should be spoken.

By now Miss Butland's days with the mobile unit were coming to an end, her work with the 'Freak Unit' was over. On 30 September 1944 she said goodbye to No.1 Mobile Military Hospital. She was posted to a general hospital in Sicily, but once again military bureaucracy proved very trying for her. For a short time, she was not allowed to sail on her own, but in Naples she received movement orders, which stated that she 'travel by road'. Despite having gone through circles to secure a flight to Sicily, the flight was cancelled immediately because, on seeing the order, the officer in charge refused to let her board saying 'Flying is not stipulated in these orders!' She pointed out that Sicily was an island and the only way to get there was to fly, but this was to no avail. Miss

Butland then had to commandeer an ambulance and drive herself twenty miles to seek permission. On 10 December 1944 she was again en route for Naples, but this time on a ship bound for home. She was then despatched to Ireland on a psychiatric course in preparation for a posting in Bangalore, India, assisting Burmese patients who needed psychiatric treatment.

Following this brief stay in India, Miss Butland returned to civilian life where she had to begin piecing together her nursing career. Firstly as assistant matron in the General Hospital, Stockport, then Bristol, and then at Gravesend for two years. Miss Butland realized she was not accumulating a pension, so she looked around for a matron post. She gained the appointment of Matron at the General Hospital, Workington, in Cumbria, where she built up the hospital from seventy beds to over two hundred. The hospital had originally started out with only six beds, built on the top of a slag-heap. It was built for the miners and they paid sixpence a week to ensure that they would always have a bed and did not have to pay any doctors' fees.

Miss Butland's responsibilities grew again. As well as the general hospital, she became responsible for a thirty-bed maternity hospital, a tuberculosis hospital, a training school and two small hospitals in the region. Her nursing and organizational experiences were now available to a wider community. Having witnessed a great deal of change during her years of nursing, especially during the Second World War, she brought these experiences to her work.

It was a period of rapid social evolution, which had raised women's expectations. With this change, a new breed of woman was entering the work-force; she was more headstrong and worldly. Whereas the rules of the nursing profession had remained immutable up until the war and students were still being 'kept in line', the principles set out by Florence Nightingale were being challenged. Even the role of matron was beginning to be challenged. Reflecting on the changes she has seen over the years, Miss Butland accepts that change is important and that nursing must move on.

However, she does not like the modern idea of portraying matrons as dragons. 'It is very wrong, they were nothing of the sort. You got the occasional one who might be a bit fiery but dragons, no! You get that with anything, teachers, doctors and bosses in industry.' She relates a pre-war story where a nurse ignored the nursing home rules and, as a punishment, was put in charge of switching all the lights out at night; it worked, her behaviour improved! Another nurse who also defied the rules was dealt with in a different way; a student, she had 'beautiful hair, beautiful'. The students wore caps and they were not allowed to have their hair hanging down. Miss Butland had often told this nurse to put it up in a net, but she always ignored her. She sent for the nurse one morning and told her either to go to the hairdresser's and get it cut or, if not, always to wear it up in a net. Miss Butland then told her that if she did not comply, she would get a pair of scissors and cut it off herself, and that it would not be as good a job as her hairdresser could do. She asked the nurse to come and see her the next morning, but the nurse didn't come! Miss Butland sent for her and saw that the nurse had not had it cut, so she sat her in a chair and cut it. Not too badly, she added. A long time after that incident, she met her again and the nurse said to Miss Butland, 'Do you know, Matron, that was the best thing you could have done for me when you cut my hair. It was then that I realized how unnecessarily rebellious I had been.' Miss Butland recalls, 'We were the authority and, having made a decision, we had to follow it through. You could do that then. Can you imagine that today?'

Miss Butland retired from nursing at the age of sixty in 1963. Not yet ready to rest, for many years she was the companion of the mother of a family in the Highlands of Scotland. She remembers it as a very regal place with a mile-long drive, servants, butlers and excellent hospitality.

Having attended the parade of Dunkirk Veterans in 1998, Miss Butland's one remaining ambition, at the age of ninety-eight, is to gain a room on a lower floor of the house where she now resides. 'For the time when I may be less able to climb four flights of stairs four times a day.'

Note

1 General Montgomery insisted that 'medical efficiency [is] a vital ingredient in maintaining morale, and morale is the big thing in war; that it is vital for commanders to 'take personal responsibility for prompt air evacuation, good surgical teams, and availability of blood transfusion, and nurses well forward'. Hamilton, N., *Monty: Master of the Battlefield, 1942-1944* (Hamish Hamilton Ltd., London, 1983).

VIII

A Changing War Role for QARNNS Matrons

In the early nineteenth century, the Falkland Islands became a British colony. The main islands are East and West Falkland, with their dependencies the South Georgia and South Sandwich islands. The Argentinians named the islands the Islas Malvinas, and have long laid claim to them, although the population is almost entirely of British origin. On 2 April 1982, Argentina invaded the islands. Attempts to reach a diplomatic solution failed and a task force was sent from the United Kingdom, initially capturing South Georgia on 25 April.

Faced with a situation where casualties were expected and no land facility would be available, a floating medical service was the only alternative. Hospital ships have a long history of supporting foreign campaigns and the Falklands campaign was no exception. The ship was to be manned by experienced medical and nursing staff.

On 6 April 1982, Miss Edith Meiklejohn (later Curson), Deputy Matron of Royal Naval Hospital Haslar attended a management meeting with the Medical Officer-in-Charge to discuss the medical and nursing response to the potential conflict. They faced three initial nursing problems: first, the choice of nursing staff and skills required; second, the resultant depletion of ward staff from both RNH Haslar and RNH Stonehouse at Plymouth; and third, deciding upon which wards would have to close. By the end of the meeting Edith Meiklejohn knew she was to head the nursing team as matron.

Edith Meiklejohn started her nursing career at the Western Infirmary, Glasgow, in 1953, qualifying for her SRN in 1956. From this time, until she joined the Queen Alexandra's Royal Naval Nursing Service (QARNNS), she was developing her career opportunities through a variety of courses including parts I & II Midwifery, and an Operating Theatre Techniques course. Her QARNNS career spanned from 1962 until her retirement at the rank of Principal Nursing Officer in 1983, when she was awarded the Royal Red Cross. Her posts had ranged from Nursing Sister to Deputy Matron-in-Chief.

Edith had three days to sort out her own affairs; to shop for suitable things to take with her, arrange her uniform, inform her family, pay the bills via the bank, and arrange for someone to look after the house and garden. The uncertainty of not knowing what transport she would be using, or when and where she would be going, did not help her with these decisions. She joined the *Canberra* on 9 April, met the rest of the medical team, and was immediately thrown into an endless round of planning wards and sorting out equipment and stores. There seemed to be a never-ending necessity to move stores from one place to another. Apart from the medical and nursing teams there were two thousand troops, and because the ship was carrying these troops, the *Canberra* had been excluded as a hospital ship under the Geneva Convention. They sailed on 9 April to the sound of Royal Marine and Parachute Regiment bands playing ashore, with fireworks, hooting cars, ship horns and flashing car lights along the quayside. 'A most amazing noise and sight, and very emotional, the uncertainty of what and where we were headed, very much in everyone's thoughts!'

On Thursday, 15 April 1982, thirty-seven QARNNS officers and ratings quietly flew out from RAF Brize Norton to Gibraltar to join the British Peninsular and Oriental Steamship Company liner the SS *Uganda*. The nurses found that the Hercules was the most uncomfortable type of plane to fly in, especially as the planes were overstocked with as much equipment as could physically be fitted on board. 'The "heads" was literally a bucket with a curtain draped round it. There were drinks, but we avoided them so we would not have to use it.' Box meals were provided. Five hours was a long time; able to stand and stretch but not move around, by the time they landed they were all tired, aching and dehydrated. It was described by all as a grim start.

On board the Hercules was Superintending Nursing Sister Julia Massey. Just days before, Miss Massey had been on a ward round at RNH Stonehouse, Plymouth with matron, when there was a telephone call from the MoD in London asking for six more nurses and sisters to join the task force. Matron promptly asked her if she would go, and when she agreed two days later, she was replaced on the ward and was off. 'Matron could do that!' She joined other medical officers, nursing sisters and QARNNS, male royal naval nurses, and medical assistants, physiotherapists, radiologists, and pharmacy dispensers. There was the opportunity to develop a team spirit as they worked side by side in general preparations and lectures, and when they were being kitted out.

In previous conflicts civilian ships, referred to as 'ships taken up from the trade' (STUFT), were converted into hospital ships such as the SS *Uganda*. The Royal Navy had requisitioned the SS *Uganda* from its civilian duties in Naples to serve as the hospital ship in support of military services for the expected conflict in the Falklands. P&O maintained the SS *Uganda* as an educational cruise ship for children. With its dormitory layout it was thought most suitable to convert to hospital accommodation, but it had to be fitted out within days. The main structural change was the helicopter platform added to the upper deck, and a new ramp to the lower deck for transportation of patients from the flight deck to the hospital area. The ship was emblazoned with red crosses in keeping with Geneva Convention rules.

A few days were spent in Gibraltar for the refit, with the dockyard workers doing an amazing job in just three or four days. A lot of the furnishings were taken out, and the wood panelling boarded up. In the ward below the flight deck, the panelling was taken back to the bulkheads in readiness. Store supplies were intended for a field hospital and were not adequate for keeping patients in a hospital for a considerable period of time. They had shortages of basic nursing equipment such as weights for traction, bedpans and thermometers. Further stores were requisitioned and flown out to Ascension Island. Miss Massey became temporary Divisional Officer responsible for the QARNNS nurses. The nurses were placed in four- and six-bedded accommodations, as were the royal naval medical assistants. The P&O staff looked after them well with stewards to clean the cabins and make the beds while they looked after the hospital.

The SS *Uganda* sailed from Gibraltar on 14 April. While sailing south, the nurses worked with the medical staff sorting out the allocation of areas into wards. One ward at the stern was named 'Seaview Ward' because of the lovely view, but the windows were soon to be boarded up. This was to be the high dependency ward where Miss Massey was to be in charge of the nursing for forty-four beds. Forward from there was a triage area and the ramp from the upper deck came into this area to transfer the patients down. In the triage area, as its name suggests, the patients would very quickly be assessed and prioritized to see where in the hospital they should go. Further forward were the operating theatres with two operating tables; these were sometimes in use for fourteen hours a day. They also had to set up the autoclaves in that area. The hairdressing department became the radiography department, with the X-ray machine just outside. The cocktail bar became the packing area for the theatres and wards. There was a pharmacy area and a smaller area for the intensive care ward with twenty-two beds. On the right was the music room, which became the ward room for the officers; this was planned for and later converted to a ward for burns care. The nurses became experts at improvising, and inventing things to make equipment work. They had no cupboard space at all and eventually managed to get hold of the crates that the theatre tables and X-ray equipment had come in and they lashed these to the deck to store equipment.

Matron Meiklejohn arrived at Ascension Island at 07.45 on Tuesday 20 April and spent the next week not being sure whether she was to stay with the *Canberra* or be transferred to the *Uganda*. On 27 April she was informed that she was to take over as matron of the hospital ship facility on the SS *Uganda*. Two days later she said her farewells and transferred by helicopter to SS *Uganda*.

Fresh water was a problem because the SS *Uganda* was, in peace time, never more than four days away from a port, so during a war, when it had to remain at sea for longer, there was a terrible water shortage. They had to get used to taking thirty-second showers. At Ascension Island, desalination units arrived – these were fitted to the upper deck and affectionately known as 'Kariba' and 'Niagara'. Asked by Matron, on a very cold day, how they were performing, the Lieutenant Commander (E) replied that they were chucking out 'b— ice cubes'.

For Matron and her staff it was a journey into a relatively unknown area. The war role of QARNNS nursing staff would have been introduced at various courses and training sessions within the royal naval medical services. Up until the Falkland Islands crisis however, the focus of any conflict was always the Cold War areas in the north, not hostilities in the South Atlantic Ocean.

The war role of the Royal Marine Bandsmen was as stretcher-bearers. The stretchers were canvas and the marines had to manoeuvre the patients out of the helicopters and down a steep ramp into the triage area where beds were set up. Once the patients had been assessed, unless they were able to walk, the marines had to carry them on stretchers either to the intensive care ward, down into Seaview, or into the dormitories. This was an extraordinarily difficult exercise to perform on a rolling ship. The nurses also taught the marines some basic nursing duties, such as washing patients, taking temperatures and lifting. Everyone was trained intensively.

Miss Meiklejohn attended heads of department meetings every evening, some of which, of course, could be quite rancorous with everyone fighting for staff for their particular areas. Staff shortage was quite acute. These meetings increased in frequency to twice a day when they were nearing the Falklands. Matron and the medical officers started to organize hospital admission and disposal exercises, practising the reception of casualties and how they would be moved around the hospital. It was still difficult for the nurses to believe that war would be declared. They used to congregate at about twelve o'clock and listen to the BBC World Service, this being the only way they could know what was happening. It all seemed so normal. After being in the exclusion zone for a week they were then told to go right down to the Falklands. It was a calm night, the sky was clear and the stars were at their brightest. On deck, Miss Meiklejohn and Miss Massey felt a sense of anticipation tinged with anxiety, 'At last it was happening, we were off.' Like all the nurses, the worst thing for them had been the waiting. 'Was all that practice going to pay off, would the hospital systems work, have we covered every eventuality?' they wondered.

Staff nicknamed the SS *Uganda*, 'NOSH', because it was the naval ocean-going surgical hospital and the navy's own equivalent to MASH (Mobile Army Surgical Hospital). They did actually write 'NOSH' on the flight deck. They were joined by three royal naval hydrography ships, HMS *Hydra*, HMS *Hecla* and HMS *Herald*, adapted as hospital and ambulance ships, and these transported the patients from SS *Uganda* to Montevideo. It took them five days to get there and then five days to come back. The SS *Uganda* was affectionately known as 'Mother Hen', and the three ships were her chicks.

Miss Meiklejohn spent these days in an increasing number of meetings: the Medical Officer-in-Charge in the morning, and the heads of department in the evening. Getting to know, and working with, her staff was a high priority. Because some of the nurses were very young (the youngest was twenty), there were times when things could be difficult for them. There were other issues for matron to sort out as well, such as problems for the nurses accepting the concept of Triage, plus the inevitable overcrowding of wards and low levels of staff.

How to dispose of the dead was also discussed, but in the event only three servicemen died on board and they were returned to the Falkland Islands to be buried there.

On 4 April, HMS *Sheffield* was attacked and sunk in a surprise attack by the Argentinian Air Force. In her diary of Wednesday 12 May, Miss Meiklejohn reported the first four casualties received from the attack on HMS *Sheffield*: a Petty Officer who was badly burned and three junior ratings who were not so severely burned. All of the men were in shock. Miss Massey observed, 'It was so sad. They talked of little presents and things they had brought back for their wives and children, all lost. It was quite poignant, hearing them talk about quite simple things, little things. They were very upset.' When casualties started to arrive in large numbers, the value of the matron role became apparent. She was able to have a complete overview of the situation and had the authority to move her staff to areas that were experiencing undue pressure.

In the Seaview area that Miss Massey managed were the patients with shrapnel, gunshot and blast injuries. Much of the nursing was orthopaedic work because of the damaged limbs, and the nurses had the added worry of infection getting into open wounds and, more importantly, into bones. Miss Massey explained, 'With gunshot wounds there's always an entry and an exit, and sometimes there are multiple exit wounds, particularly on buttocks and limbs. These wounds got packed but remained open.' The treatment of wounds has been very well tried and tested. Guidelines were laid down in the Second World War as to how wounds should be treated, and these have not changed greatly. War wounds have to have any debris removed and the dead skin cut away from around them, and then the wounds are cleaned and packed so that granulation takes place from below; therefore such wounds are not sutured.

Most of the casualties had emergency surgery ashore at Ajax Bay, which was the medical facility on the Falklands, before coming to the SS *Uganda* some twenty-four hours later. They had received excellent treatment. Some of these men would go to theatre on the ship again that same day, or

certainly within twenty-four hours. They were given intravenous antibiotics and analgesics, and would go to theatre
every two or three days to have their wounds repacked. Very
little wound dressing was done on the ward because the dressings were massive, requiring 'the boys' to be given anaesthetics. Because of the problems associated with giving people
numerous anaesthetics, it proved to be quite an interesting
time because different anaesthetics were used on different
days: on some days the patients would be wide awake very
quickly, on other days they would remain very sleepy; some
days they would cry a lot, and on other days they could get
very amorous. This was very challenging for the nurses.

Miss Meiklejohn and her nursing staff had enormous
respect for these young men. They described working with
servicemen as a unique experience because the men were of a
limited age group, they were fit and they all wanted to get
better. 'It was amazing how cheerful they remained and how
they just got on with things.' They would have to go to X-ray
then to theatre, and the next morning they would be sitting up
in bed cheerfully washing. The soldiers must have been so
relieved that they had got to the ship since they must have had
a terribly uncomfortable twenty-four hours since being
injured. Being in a bed between clean sheets, having hot food
provided and having female nurses around would all add to
their initial recovery. The nurses noted another difference
between nursing servicemen and civilians. 'Servicemen are
used to living with [each other]. They are not embarrassed or
coy, and they have this buddy-buddy care. So they do help
each other.' When fit enough, patients were moved to the
dormitories; each morning there was a 'clear out' to make
beds available for the new casualties coming on that day.

The ship's log for 25 May reports the SS *Uganda* being
buzzed by two Argentinian Sky Hawks. They hurtled down
either side of the ship, and the noise was tremendous. This
made everyone nervous as they realized just how vulnerable
they were. Five Sky Hawks also buzzed them on 28 May.
They were protected under the Geneva Convention and as
Argentina had signed up to this, it was hoped they would

follow the Convention Rules.

For Miss Meiklejohn, Saturday 12 June was a low day. She recorded in her diary:

> HMS *Glamorgan* has been hit, will all this ever end?
>
> The major attack by our troops commenced at 0200. Argentinians say that their hospital ship has been attacked, Members of the International Red Cross on board at the time were able to refute this statement. We had eighty-five casualties in during the day so were really overloaded. *Hecla* was able to take seventy-one on board which helped, there are still patients on the deck, everywhere is overflowing. The troops are in a good position round Port Stanley. It is estimated that we shall receive about a hundred casualties in the next two days. The patients who are able help others with feeding, visits to the heads [toilets] and with washing.

By 28 June, the conflict situation had deteriorated further with more casualties. At this point many casualties were sleeping on mattresses on the deck. Matron Meiklejohn noted:

> Started off with a quiet morning then all hell breaks loose. We were able to transfer forty-four patients to *Hecla* including some Argentinians. This was done in a force ten with fifty-foot waves, the pilots doing a marvellous job. During the day we had thirty-seven casualties from 45 Commando and the Paras, plus others. Three are badly injured and two go for immediate surgery. Everybody worked hard and well.

For the casualties, especially those with fractures, the constant pitching of the ship in bad weather caused even greater distress.

The longest stretch Miss Meiklejohn allowed nurses to be on duty for was four hours; they would have time to eat and sleep and then go back to work. This did cause some grumbles, but Matron felt a reversion to eight-hour shifts would be too tiring at sea and, as the whole ship was turned into a hospital, there was little to do except work, eat, and sleep. At the hospital's busiest, the nurses could be up day and night. When the ship encountered bad weather, the staff were constantly fighting seasickness caused by the rolling of the ship, so the watch times were reduced to alleviate this problem. An additional problem was sleep being interrupted by constant tannoy messages. When it announced 'Hands to flying stations', they knew the helicopters were bringing casualties.

Matron's diary for Monday 31 May explains the situation encountered on entering San Carlos Bay, with its very rugged scenery.

Thirty-seven casualties today; again many very seriously injured, eighteen of them Argentinian. The latter were very dirty and hungry, suffering from hypothermia and very bad trench foot, they were also extremely frightened.

An extra twelve nursing staff drafted to NOSH making a great difference. They had to move the fit Argentineans from D-Deck to B-Deck, as it was impossible to get the stretchers down the gangways. They had one hundred and eighty-seven patients. One Royal Marine had his life saved when an enemy bullet hit his army manual in his pocket.

1 June: been on board *Uganda* since 29 April – thirty-two days, feel as though I have always been here and there has been no other life! Thankful for all the letters and good wishes from my family and colleagues, and for the companionship of the people on board.

Extra help did arrive with staff joining from SS *Canberra* because their medical facility was not after all taking as many patients as had been originally envisaged. Often some of the crew from other ships came and helped; the cooks and stewards particularly liked to help out. Some of the officers of the SS *Uganda* would help, including one officer who used to come to the wards every morning at about six o'clock.

They were constantly short of syringes, the same syringe

having to be used for twenty-four hours, but they had plenty of needles. Because they were constantly in touch with the other ships (the 'three chicks'), there were no great problems with medications although the types of antibiotics, analgesics and night sedatives used had to be changed regularly because of increasing demand for them and an intermittent supply. Another acute problem arose with blood for transfusion. Having 'long life' blood on board solved the initial problems about supply, but then the blood started to deteriorate and lose its clotting factor. On one occasion they called over the tannoy for donors to go to the theatre to provide fresh blood. Miss Massey, because she had one of the blood groups needed, volunteered and the next day 'reminded the young soldier who was the recipient to be very careful with it!'

The ship was lit up the whole time, which was another requirement of the Geneva Convention. They could not have coded signals to the ship, because everything had to be open. Every evening they would sail away from the Falklands in order to use the desalination plants to make the fresh water supply; they would also get rid of the 'gash' (refuse) into deeper water. Early in the morning they would sail back again and by about eight o'clock they would be in Falkland Sound. From reports it does seem that they did upset a number of Royal Navy ships because they were so brightly lit, but they quickly moved off. There was concern among naval ships that the SS *Uganda* might get hit if the Navy themselves were being targeted, so they wanted to keep well away. As it was they thought the SS *Uganda* was very lucky not to have been hit.

The wards had no privacy for the patients who were bedridden. Miss Massey pointed out that it is not so bad for men because they can use bottles to urinate in, but that there was an awful lot of use of bedpans in the middle of the night. She thought being servicemen they would get on with it, but that civilians would have found difficulty coping. Of course they didn't have the quality of bedpan-washers on board ship that they had in hospitals. There was a Heath Robinson bedpan washer set up on each ward, plumbed by a hose into the piped water supply. To wash the bedpans out they were given great big rubber gloves. Compromising was the order of the day. Even the weights for orthopaedic traction were plastic lemonade bottles filled with water and hung at the ends of beds, and not proper weights. Something else learned by all was the essential need to prioritize. Certainly the administration of drugs and antibiotics took much longer than had previously been experienced, sometimes up to two hours. All the patients were on antibiotics, some via an intravenous drip, others by intramuscular injection.

The first Argentinian soldiers who came on board were kept for about three weeks. Their own hospital ship system was not organized at that time, but by the end of the conflict they had three hospital ships and SS *Uganda* had to meet up regularly with them to transfer the Argentinian patients over. It was very obvious which soldiers were conscripts and which were the regular soldiers because the conscripts had no identification discs around their necks. Initially the men were healthy, but hungry. Some of them were obviously very frightened, and it was evident that most of them did not know where they were, that they were at the Falklands. The Argentinean and English patients were in the same wards. There was no obvious animosity between them, but one Argentinian officer, an air force pilot who had been ejected from his aircraft, proved to be a very arrogant man and totally refused to help translate for his soldiers – the nurses found this upsetting.

The Argentinian patients were treated in the same way as the British patients, with the same treatments, food and everything else. They suffered mainly blast injuries and gunshot wounds towards the end of the fighting. There were also problems with trench-foot and gangrene caused by the cold and wet conditions, and there was evidence of neglect by individual soldiers themselves. In the last few days, six Argentineans were admitted who had obviously been neglecting themselves. The nursing staff felt they had done this deliberately, to be taken out of the fighting. They had horrendous gangrene of their toes and feet. They suspected that one of them had deliberately shot himself in the foot. They were only kept on board for a few hours and then transferred to their hospital ship, and probably ended up having bilateral amputations, which the staff felt was very sad.

Miss Massey reflected on a nurse's role nursing the enemy under the Geneva Convention. 'The requirement is that they nurse the enemy, a nurse is there to aid the sick and injured. Of course, the soldiers and sailors in the war are also aware of the Geneva Convention, and that they also have a duty to look after the enemy. There was no animosity towards the Argentinians as individuals, and everyone was aware that there may be British casualties in Argentine hospital ships.'

The SS *Uganda* met up quite regularly with one of the Argentinian hospital ships, the *Bahia Paraiso*, often exchanging drugs and treatment advice, doctor to doctor. Miss Meiklejohn gave the Argentinian medical staff quite a surprise when she was helicoptered across for a visit. 'They just did not expect a woman to be serving aboard a ship in a period of war.' Once news of the surrender became known in the middle of June it was obviously quieter. There were less casualties and, over the next week or ten days, the staff transferred all the patients over to one of the survey vessels for the journey home. The ship then had to remain on station because SS *Uganda* was to be the hospital facility for service personnel in the Falklands until the army field hospital arrived.

Shortly after the ship was decommissioned, Miss Meiklejohn reported in her diary of Wednesday 13 July:

> There was an accident at the airfield where soldiers were clearing the runway of snow when a Harrier accidentally fired its sidewinder weapon, injuring many. There are amputations and some very shocked soldiers, this on the day the Red Crosses were being painted out. So very sad. The area that had been the intensive care had been renamed Stanley Ward. It was re-opened and we were busy again. This was a bitter blow to all.

When the SS *Uganda* left the Falklands on18 July, it was a merchant ship once again. They had a quiet time sailing to

England, docking at Southampton on 9 August, which they felt was probably good as it gave them time to talk over their experiences. Miss Massey summed up the return leg of the journey in the following way: they knew what they were doing and it worked. She thinks having the three weeks between leaving the Falklands and returning to England did allow the servicemen a time for reflection and to start thinking about going home. It is believed that if people have a period of time to reflect together and talk it is beneficial. Miss Massey thought there would have been even more problems and more difficulties settling back at home if they had arrived back within a twenty-four hour period. Certainly everybody was looking forward to getting back to Southampton.

Miss Meiklejohn's report states that the treatment of casualties commenced on 12 May and continued until 13 July.

> It really was a great achievement with the organization running so successfully. The routines that were practised worked well. The greatest number of casualties in one day was 160, the injured from the RFA *Sir Galahad* and RFA *Sir Tristram*. The emergency ward was opened on that day and remained in use for three weeks ... In total there were 730 casualties received on board, of whom 159 were Argentinians, these were eventually transferred to their own hospital ships. There were three deaths on board, all British.

Of the 128 medical staff who complemented the hospital ship SS *Uganda*, forty-four were members of QARNNS. They were eventually to spend a hundred and thirteen challenging and professionally rewarding days at sea. The fifteen nursing officers and twenty-nine nurses had been admirably suited to the task they had faced. People have since asked many of the nurses if they found it traumatic nursing the war wounded. Miss Massey sums it up as follows:

> I suppose not really, because although we hadn't seen war wounds, we had seen wounds from our daily work as nurses and from accidents. So I don't think we did find it upsetting,

no, we were so busy that you really didn't have time to think about it. It is like people have said to me, 'Were you frightened of the ship being hit and [for] your own safety?' I suppose we were, but nursing has to go on twenty-four hours a day.

In recognition of the exemplary effort contributed by her nurses, Matron Meiklejohn stated:

The numbers of nursing staff were barely adequate to meet the needs imposed on them. Maintaining this level of nursing care over a longer period and with such a large number of casualties would have stretched any nurse beyond endurance and many beyond their capabilities however willing, but the nurses on board the SS *Uganda* showed great courage, resourcefulness and dedication. They worked exceptionally hard under the most trying conditions, coping with appalling injuries the like of which the majority had not seen before. The mental anguish of seeing such young men so badly injured was felt by all.

IX
Living on a Knife-Edge

Less than nine years after the Falklands War, a Matron was once again to lead a nursing team into a war situation – the Gulf War.

Miss Gillian Comrie ARRC completed her general and midwifery training at the Royal London Hospital between 1964 and 1969, and joined Queen Alexandra's Royal Naval Nursing Service in 1970. During almost twenty-six years of service she held a variety of appointments, both in the UK and abroad, and was promoted to Chief Nursing Officer in 1989. Following her service in the Gulf as Matron, she was appointed Matron to Royal Naval Hospital, Plymouth. Her last appointments in QARNNS were in the Royal Navy Headquarters where she was deputy to Director Naval Nursing Services/Matron-in-Chief QARNNS, and then she was the In-service Training Officer responsible for all QARNNS qualified nurse specialist training and Naval General Training. Miss Comrie left QARNNS in 1996 with the rank of Commander.

In August 1990 Saddam Hussein invaded Kuwait. Within a few weeks it became obvious that British forces would be involved and that medical and nursing teams would be required to support the various military units deployed. In previous conflicts where nursing support was required to cover the deployed RN ships, civilian ships, referred to as 'ships taken up from trade' (STUFT), were converted into hospital ships such as SS *Uganda* in the Falklands War. In the Gulf War a new concept was introduced, in the form of a Primary Casualty Receiving Ship (PCRS). It was proposed to put a purpose-built hospital unit inside a Royal Fleet Auxiliary (RFA) ship. This hospital unit was to be in 'collective protection', which meant that in the event of nuclear, biological or chemical attack the hospital unit could 'close down' thus protecting its environment and the patients and staff within. The nominated ship was to be RFA *Argus*, whose peacetime role was that of Helicopter Training Ship for the RN Fleet Air Arm because it had a flight deck that accommodated six Sea King helicopters. The helicopters would be used to transport patients from the field of battle, be it land or sea, to the PCRS. The hospital unit was to be below the flight deck in the foremost hangar of four, with its own helicopter lift, which would be used for the movement of patients from the flight deck to the hospital.

The hospital was intended to contain one hundred beds. Following various layout trials and exercises during passage to the Gulf, the following allocation of beds was decided: ten Intensive Care beds (ITU), fourteen High Dependency (HDU) and seventy-six Low Dependency beds (LDU). Apart from the ward areas, the hospital was to contain two operating theatres – one with two tables for major surgery, with anaesthetic and recovery areas, and the other for minor surgery, which also was used for physiotherapy treatments. There would also be a reception area and a small galley. There was an autoclave capable of running on liquid or solid fuel, gas or electricity; this was under the direction of the theatre superintendent. Throughout the hospital there were seven toilets and a bank of wash-basins. There was only one decent-sized cupboard inside the hospital and this was soon converted into an X-ray developing room. Large pieces of equipment were stowed outside the hospital, lashed to the hangar bulkhead; other items were stowed under the beds in large boxes which were fixed to the beds with tape or string. Bedside lockers were also used for the storage of medical items. Within the hospital there were various items of equipment for basic haematological and biochemical assessment. The nursing staff was to total forty-two nursing personnel comprising one matron, four operating theatre nursing officers and a further five to run ITU/HDU, LDU and the Reception area; five senior rate nurses, and twenty-seven junior rate nurses and medical assistants. This nursing team was to be made up largely from female personnel.

In her normal role, RFA *Argus* accommodated approximately a hundred and twenty personnel. During active service, additional personnel were needed to enable the ship to fulfil her role. The additional personnel consisted of a Royal Navy detachment to assist with the day-to-day running of the ship, an RN Fleet Air Arm squadron to fly and maintain the helicopters, a Royal Marines Band detachment to act as stretcher bearers (all of these marines were qualified in advanced first aid and trained in basic nursing skills on arrival in the Gulf), and the hospital medical, nursing, technical and administrative staff, in excess of 400 personnel.

As Deputy Matron at Royal Naval Hospital Haslar it was no surprise to Commander Comrie that she would be appointed matron of the PCRS and she was happy to assume this responsibility, particularly as she had remained in the UK during the Falklands War. Then the medical and nursing staff were nominated, about which Commander Comrie notes: 'One interesting aspect of the nursing team was that there was a reversal of the conventional role where the wife stayed at home and the husband goes to war. This time in some cases the husbands were left at home and the wife went off to the war.'

The total hospital team was to consist of QARNNS nurses, royal naval doctors, physiotherapists, radiographers, operating theatre staff, pharmacist dispenser, laboratory technicians plus a hospital padre. Also, lessons being learned from the Falklands War, for the first time a psychiatric team joined the group. As the appointed matron to the PCRS, Commander Comrie would be responsible for appropriate levels and standards of nursing care, the day-to-day running of the hospital ward areas, and the general housekeeping of the unit. She also had to make certain that at all times nursing teams would be available and prepared to nurse whatever situation confronted them. With the Falklands War having happened less than nine years previously, she had the experience of nursing colleagues to draw upon. She did this before joining *Argus*, speaking to as many nursing personnel as possible, from all levels of seniority, who had served on SS *Uganda*. The information she gained was of great importance and was taken into account when organizing the various teams, duties and routines.

This team's situation was to be very different from that of staff on previous hospital ships. They did not come under the terms of the Geneva Convention, and the staff, when not caring for the patients, would have to be involved in 'whole ship' duties, along with all other RN personnel on board. These duties included lifting and shifting general stores from shore to ship or around the ship, cleaning routines in other areas outside the hospital domain, and being a member of duty watch and emergency teams.

The nursing officer appointed as operating theatre Superintendent and Commander Comrie visited HMNB Plymouth, where RFA *Argus* was undergoing conversion. Comrie needed to familiarize herself with the layout of the ship so that she could brief staff as thoroughly as possible; she also needed to see the hospital unit and accommodation. A 'twenty-seven man' mess had been allocated to the junior rate female personnel. This consisted of a sleeping area of bunks in tiers of three divided by limited personal lockers, plus a seating area for approximately fifteen people. With such limited space nurses were able to bring with them little more than their uniforms. Everything had to be stowed and secured safely; any item not secured properly could prove hazardous during ship manoeuvres and 'action stations'. The nearest area for ablutions designated to them was inadequate for their number and several decks up from their mess deck. Commander Comrie had to negotiate with the Chief Officer to resolve the situation, and it was marginally improved prior to sailing. She proposed that the PCRS Officers' and Senior Rates' ablutions areas be made available to the junior rate nurses at two fixed times each day. Consequently nurses were allocated to specific areas at these times. Although not ideal, it became a workable solution.

With PCRS personnel nominated by early October, Commander Comrie briefed all nursing staff in RNH Haslar and arranged the same brief for RNH Plymouth. Mindful of the shortage of stowage areas, she proposed that all nursing personnel take two paperback books with them, thus providing an initial library for them to draw upon. Staff were also advised to take a swimming kit, and no more than two civilian casual outfits in case the opportunity arose to go ashore. The rest of the locker space available to them would be taken up with uniforms and essential personal items. The majority also took with them small pieces of fine embroidery or canvas work.

Additional naval training was programmed for and undertaken prior to sailing; this included damage control, firefighting and familiarization with the ship. Staff were also issued with operational uniforms, protection and personal equipment. Members of the team were allowed a few days of additional leave to enable them to get their personal administration in order and say farewell to relatives and friends. Although Commander Comrie was aware of the nurses' additional qualifications, she was not aware of their nursing experience, so she requested that they all supply her with this in order that she might place each member of staff in the most appropriate working area. Nurses were thus divided into teams in which they remained for the total deployment. There were some male nursing personnel allocated between the teams to provide additional 'muscle' to assist with lifting and shifting.

When planning the nursing watch system, it was important to take account not only of the needs of patients, but also the needs of staff and the ship's routine. As some form of hot meal was available at six-hourly intervals it was essential that hospital staff work around their hours because staffing numbers were not sufficient to release staff for meals during their watch. In addition, hospital staff would have to take the patients' meals from the galley to the hospital when coming on duty, and return dirty cutlery and plates when going off duty. They did have microwaves and kettles in the hospital for the provision of hot drinks and for warming-up food, but these were not adequate for preparing main meals. Commander Comrie decided that a six-hour watch system would be introduced. It was unrealistic for nurses to work six-hours on duty then six-off like the rest of the ship, so she introduced a three-watch system for nursing personnel. This would allow six hours on duty, followed by six hours' sleep, and then six hours' stand-by time, enabling her to call additional staff from the standing watch if required in the hospital during heavy periods of work, thus protecting those on the sleeping watch. This was why she made the initially unpopular decision to allocate junior rate nurses' bunk spaces to the Mess; it would mean that when additional nursing personnel were required in the hospital, they could be called with the minimum of fuss, not disturbing those on the sleeping watch. It was envisaged that additional nursing staff would certainly be required when receiving casualties.

The majority of staff were to work in the Intensive Care and High Dependency units and, when not receiving patients, the nursing staff in the Reception area would assist in these two units. There was minimal staffing in the Low Dependency area as the patients were more able to look after themselves. They could also assist their fellow patients, as was proven on board SS *Uganda* during the Falklands War. The plan was that during times of action the ship would manoeuvre close to the 'front line' and receive casualties via the helicopters or boats, using the ship's crane and a cradle to lift the latter from the water. If required, casualties would be processed through the decontamination unit on the flight deck before entering the hospital through the Triage area, using the Advanced Trauma Life Support (ATLS) system. Once the hospital unit was full, the ship would sail out of the war zone. During this period patients would undergo whatever treatment/care was appropriate. At an identified safe area the casualties would be offloaded to an airfield, and flown to a military hospital before repatriation to the UK. RFA *Argus* would then return to the frontline and, during this return trip, the hospital would be cleaned, re-stocked and re-equipped, and the staff would rest.

RFA *Argus* sailed from Plymouth on 23 October 1990, along with some of the civilian dockyard workers who were completing work on the hospital. They were flown home when passing Gibraltar. Stores continued to arrive throughout the ten weeks prior to the commencement of hostilities; these ten weeks were full of unpacking and assembling equipment for the hospital. It was rather like Christmas – they knew what was wanted, but did not know exactly what had arrived until they opened the various boxes and crates, getting very excited when a 'high-powered' or long-awaited item arrived. At the onset of hostilities all required medical stores and equipment had arrived.

When they departed the UK it was thought that the war would start in mid November, hence the speedy departure, but the deadline kept moving and eventually war commenced on the night of 16 January 1991. In the intervening weeks they trained and took part in various exercises within the hospital ship and with the Royal Navy and NATO Task Force. They prepared and trained for all sorts of eventualities, ranging from a hospital unit full of patients suffering all types of illness and injury, to a civilian evacuation scenario where several hundred people would be transported in *Argus* from their home to a place of safety. They fine-tuned their procedures, and designed and commissioned additional pieces of equipment to assist with working routines, mindful that everything had to be secured for safety. They were able to visit army field hospitals and also the United States hospital ships, *Comfort* and *Mercy*, both of which remained in the southern Gulf during the war.

Floating mines were seen in the Gulf in mid-January, so all ships had to be additionally vigilant. The ship's helicopter squadron was immediately enhanced with two additional helicopters, and Royal Marine bandsmen were to perform lookout duties on deck. Commander Comrie proposed that the junior rate nurses could also undertake these duties when the hospital did not have patients. This would not only assist the RM watch rota, but would also give the nurses a non-nursing ship responsibility and some space in the fresh air, a rare commodity within a crowded ship. The need for such vigilance was brought home very forcefully when two American warships hit floating mines. One ship was severely damaged, resulting in the hospital unit receiving three patients, one of whom had major head injuries which required urgent attention in the operating theatre. These were the only 'war-injured' patients they treated in the hospital; all the other patients, of which there were over a hundred, suffered from the more usual, day-to-day ailments such as appendicitis, burns, strains, twisted and torn muscles, broken bones and a variety of other minor medical conditions.

It was a frustrating time. From the onset of hostilities the nurses awoke to go on duty prepared to deal with patients with all types of injuries. They would arrive in the hospital to find it in a similar state to how they left it twelve hours before; they undertook their six-hour watch in a state of readiness, checking all equipment and thoroughly cleaning their areas; they even went off duty to bed having prepared for their next watch which could bring a full hospital unit of seriously ill and injured patients. This situation went on for forty-three days. It was an extremely frustrating time for them – they were always prepared to use their nursing skills, but they were never fully utilized. Commander Comrie considers herself fortunate that, as matron, she always had work to occupy her time, 'I do not know how I would have fared in their situation and can only admire their resolve throughout such a long and testing time.'

Suddenly the hospital team heard that they were to return to the UK within one to two days. The majority of them would fly home and RFA *Argus* would take on the role of troop carrier. The announcement produced a flurry of activity and the final hours on board passed extremely quickly, removing stores from the hospital, writing reports and getting equipment together before disembarking. The medical team left RFA *Argus* at 01:30 on 11 March 1991, fifty-five days after the onset of the Gulf War, and a hundred and thirty-nine days since leaving the UK.

We were quiet and subdued, and I think all had very mixed feelings – we were extremely glad that we had not received mass casualties at any stage during the conflict, but at the same time frustrated that we never saw the unit working to its full potential in a war situation.

X

The Cinderella Services

In the following chapter we will consider three nursing services that for years suffered from a lack of resources and isolation from society, namely mental deficiency nursing, psychiatry and workhouse infirmaries. These services were considered poor relations of general hospitals, and far removed from the more fashionable teaching hospitals. These institutions were often grim; psychiatric hospitals were frequently built way out in the country, with large walls surrounding them, and workhouse infirmaries were built generally in the poorer parts of cities. They were often feared, and even hated.

Work in these types of institutions (known for many years as the 'Cinderella Services') was hard and the nurses received little recognition. Society had very negative attitudes and showed great intolerance towards these groups of patients. The mentally ill, the mentally handicapped and the poor were treated with great suspicion and their conditions were regarded as social contagions, but through sterling work from the nursing force under the leadership of the matron in the female section, and chief male nurse (the male counterpart of Matron) in the male section, great changes were undertaken.

In institutions for the mentally handicapped and mentally ill, patients were segregated by gender, and their areas were separated by high walls. They even had separate walking areas (airing courts). This segregation was total and also applied to the staff; male nurses cared for the men, and female nurses for the women. Males and females mixed for many entertainments such as the weekly dance, cinema and Sunday Chapel; on these occasions the patients used their own (secret) sign language to communicate with each other. Gradually this segregation was lifted with the introduction of industrial workshops, education classes, and therapy departments.

At the turn of the twentieth century, patients admitted to these institutions were grouped under certain classifications. As an example of the dangers of classifying sections of the community in this way, we need look no further than here. Some of the categories used were 'Idiot', 'Imbecile' and 'Feeble-Minded' (a category that was often applied to unmarried mothers), and it took, and still is taking, a long time to fight against society's stereotypical notions about these people. 'Cretin' was the official term for a person with a thyroid deficiency.

Matron Muriel Jones would have been a success in any branch of nursing, but she deliberately chose to nurse patients known as 'subnormal'. She commenced her nurse training at the Mayday General Hospital, Croydon, in 1945. She then took midwifery training at Brighton, and then was at All Saints Hospital, Chatham. Miss Jones's parents were shocked when she chose nursing as a career, and then had a further shock when she commenced two years of training at the Bethlehem and Maudsley Hospital, London, under Matron Margaret Robinson.

Since the early centuries Bethlehem Hospital had been a leader in the field of mental illness following a Charter granted by Henry VIII. The hospital was designated for the care of 'lunatics' soon after its foundation. At that time there was no distinction made between mental illness and subnormality; such patients were regarded as born fools, an attitude dating from the reign of Edward II. Maudsley Hospital was originally a local authority hospital. When they were merged in 1948, the merger was often referred to as 'the poor, but vigorous, young bridegroom marrying the elder, well-endowed bride'.

Miss Jones wanted to travel and was interviewed at the Overseas Nursing Service. She was offered a post in Africa. As she was the only trained psychiatric nurse, her experience proved invaluable. One of the two hospitals she worked at had three thousand inmates. 'The conditions had to be seen, but I loved the work ... We had the additional chore of putting malaria tablets into patients' mouths in case the bandits had them. There was a perpetual battle against bed bugs, intestinal worms, and a fight to improve haemoglobin levels.'

On her return to England Miss Jones was appointed Assistant Matron at her original training hospital, the Bethlehem and Maudsley. While in this post, the hospital administrators proposed the opening of an experimental unit for children with mental handicaps. Miss Jones promptly took up a secondment for training in mental handicap nursing at the St Lawrence Hospital, Caterham, where Miss Tennyson was Matron. Coming from a teaching hospital it was quite a challenge. 'This was at a time when a child became sixteen years old and would be taken from the children's section across the corridor to be met by a male nurse from the adult section, and admitted to the male ward. What a sixteenth birthday!'

In 1964 there was a general financial crisis and all hospital building projects were stopped, so this project too had to be stopped. Miss Jones was still on the course at that point. She stayed at St Lawrence Hospital and took up a post as an unqualified tutor, and when the Principal Tutor left she temporarily took that post until 1972. In 1972 there was a further reorganization and the people working in the 'subnormality' field felt they had regressed to being the 'Cinderella' service all over again. 'St Lawrence had been under the direct control of the Ministry of Health, with an efficient, interested and kindly management committee.' Miss Jones was appointed Senior Nursing Officer and was responsible for fifteen wards. She retired in 1981.

Psychiatric nursing is a relatively modern concept. Before the nineteenth century mental illness was largely attributed to spiritual activity and demonic possession. Sufferers were treated with aversion and were eventually removed from society to institutions. Out of sight, out of mind! St Mary's of Bethlehem began taking lunatics in about 1377, but the curious patterns of behaviour exhibited by some patients proved highly entertaining to a voyeuristic public. Institutions encouraged freak shows where inmates were chained and left open to public ridicule and humiliation. Not until the 'Retreat' was opened in York in 1796 did a more humane approach to these people manifest itself. Understanding of mental illness gradually improved, and the old 'treatments' were questioned, but it was not until late in the nineteenth century that the practice of ducking patients in cold water and spinning them in chairs finally stopped.

Training for nurses of the mentally ill was introduced in 1891, but the General Nursing Council did not formally examine their skills until 1948. Mental health nursing was dominated by nepotism, often with generations of families working in the same hospital. Large psychiatric hospitals were self-contained and self-supporting institutions, with vast estates including a farm and staff, houses. They had their own butchers, bakers and labourers. Inmates, under the direction of the head gardener and staff, tended the farm and gardens. Separated into male and female sections, these hospitals could have thousands of beds. The male section, with a chief male nurse in charge, often enjoyed a more relaxed atmosphere, while matron, overseeing the female side, was both dreaded and respected by her patients and staff.

Shirley Metherell, a student nurse during the sixties, remembers Matron Baldwin at St James Hospital, Portsmouth: 'As students we were petrified of her, she would come round the wards regularly and everything had to be in order or there would be trouble! I think our matron was every bit as professional and formidable as any matron in a general hospital!'

In the summer of 1959, Miss K. Baldwin joined the staff of St James Hospital, Portsmouth. She was fortunate in that at the time of her arrival, money from the National Health Service had become more readily available. She used these new funds to improve living conditions for her patients and working conditions for her staff. Miss Baldwin worked directly with the architects in the planning and layout of wards and department, but rather than imposing alternative working conditions on her staff, she would always consult with them about change.

Being matron of a busy psychiatric hospital was a full-time occupation, but like many matrons, Miss Baldwin found time to be involved in the community surrounding her hospital. She was particularly interested in promoting the hospital within the community and built up valuable links with local schools. She also found time to be actively involved with the Royal College of Nursing and the National Council of Nurses. Despite the heavy workload Miss Baldwin maintained her sense of humour. Ivy McConnell relates the following story:

> Working in a psychiatric hospital you never knew what the patients would do. One day a patient was walking around with something in her shawl that she was cuddling; it was a dead rat. The pest control people were called and Matron accompanied the gentleman to the ward. We were in the dormitory having tea and toast, forbidden of course. We hurriedly pushed it under the bed only for the pest controller to say, 'We had better pull the beds out to see where they are coming from!' On seeing the toast Matron said, 'At least we are feeding them well!'

It is always an event when a matron leaves, but when Matron Baldwin left in 1967 staff saw the passing of the historic position of matron in mental hospitals. The post was to be superseded by a Chief Nursing Officer in keeping with the national trend, and in line with proposals laid down by the Ministry of Health. To the older members of staff, the new appointment was accepted with some regret, for the passing of an era is always difficult. Younger staff no doubt looked upon it as a natural progression, along with the unlocking of doors and removal of bars from the windows.

In psychiatric nursing, the segregation of male and female patients continued at many hospitals well into the 1970s. Attempts had been made to integrate the two sexes with varying success, but both the patients and the staff resisted these changes and preferred to stick to rigid, traditional practices. It was to be nurse leaders such as Chief Nurse John Greene who were prepared to stand up against outdated customs and tear down walls, both physically and metaphorically.

Mr Greene was born in County Clare, Ireland in 1916. He was one of ten children, six of whom became nurses. The family's background at Moyralla Farm with its 208 acres of land was agricultural farming and horse breeding. John grew up during a time of considerable trauma in Ireland and he also had to face illness and death early in life,. Many of his friends succumbed to tuberculosis, and his mother died following the birth of her tenth child when John was only eight. This left his father reliant on support from an aunt and cousins. At thirteen John left school to support the family farm.[1]

At eighteen Mr Greene followed his brother to England and into nursing. His first job was as a private asylum attendant at Springfield House Hospital, Bedford. There, his brother Tom was waiting to introduce him to matron. It was a very happy time, but there was none of the formal training he wanted. He took the position of probationer nurse at the Royal Eastern Counties Institution for Mental Defectives, Essex. This charitable organization promised formal tuition but delivered very little. Thrust in at the deep end he found scant training, but at least there was help from the more experienced staff.

Still in search of training, Mr Greene followed up an advertisement in the *Daily Telegraph* requesting people to apply for mental health nurse training. The assistant chief male nurse was looking for a fast bowler, a good footballer, or someone who could play a musical instrument; these were the requisite qualities for male nurses of the closed communities of asylums. Having none of these special abilities, he finally started at Herrison County Mental Hospital under Chief Male Nurse George Essex, one of the first (male) state registered general nurses to qualify when the General Nursing Council was established in 1922.

My room at Herrison was virtually a bed and very little else. The window was so high you could not see out of it. On my first day on a ward, a patient came out of a side room and started to shadow box round me, it scared me to death. When I got to know him he was fine. I was horrified at one time when I was left alone at night on a large ward with severely disturbed patients and 'bed wetters' lumped together.

At the outbreak of the Second World War, John Greene joined the Navy as a male psychiatric nurse, for the period of hostilities.

I was one of the first mentally trained nurses to join the Navy. After the basics in marching and some of the more strange rituals of service life, I joined the staff of Stonehouse Hospital, Plymouth, and promptly transferred to the Royal Naval Hospital, Chatham. Here, five other mentally trained staff and I took over the locked wards. The first thing we did was to get rid of the strait-jackets and use the padded cells to sleep in during the air raids; you never heard a thing.

Mr Greene was posted to the hospital ship *Vita*. From Alexandria they set sail for the Mediterranean, and then on to Malta and India. The following months were spent transporting patients to and from Mombasa, Colombo and Bombay. By the end of the war he was working in Ceylon caring for some of the ex-prisoners of war, captured by the Japanese. These young men were terribly traumatized by their dreadful experiences and progress was painfully slow.

Mr Greene was in Colombo when Hitler was eventually defeated and victory in Europe was declared. He had achieved the rank of petty officer, the highest rank a male nurse could reach. He was to re-enter civilian life in 1946, where his first post was as staff nurse at Herrison Hospital, Dorset, at which he had trained nearly a decade earlier. After a few months the

Chief Male Nurse took him along to the Medical Superintendent's Office, where they told him that they wanted to appoint him Assistant Chief Nurse. 'Just like that!' The hospital was still clearly divided into male and female sides; the matron was on one side, and the Chief Male Nurse on the other. Matron had the higher rank because she was head of the training school. Mr Greene was then appointed Deputy Chief Male Nurse at the progressive Moorhaven Hospital, Plymouth. A reference, dated 23 January 1948, from Dr Hunter Gillier, Deputy Medical Officer, Crichton Royal Hospital, Dumfries, a psychiatrist he had worked closely with at Chatham, already indicates the potential in a reference for Mr Greene.

> My daily work brought me into the closest contact with him [John Greene], and my early impressions of his high worth were consolidated over the years until I found I could leave him to carry out the most responsible and difficult duties in the sure knowledge that they would be quietly and meticulously performed ... It is difficult to write of him without using superlatives that may seem fulsome ... I conclude by saying that he can be recommended for the most senior position in his profession. ...

After eighteen months John Greene was appointed Chief Male Nurse.

> Now Matron and I were equals, making for a very democratic hospital. The male side was probably a little more relaxed under me than the female side under Matron, but only to a certain extent. When I went round the wards I would expect, and would receive, respect for my position. I did have some very good assistants. When we advertised for an assistant post, we had over two hundred applicants. It was after the war, with many men coming out of the forces with ambitions.

One year, when the medical superintendent was on holiday, Mr Greene had the airing court walls knocked down on both the female and male side. These were areas where patients could exercise and where the nursing staff could observe their behaviour. The walls were high, preventing any attempts to escape. The early 1970s saw the demolition of all airing court walls. John reported, 'When the medical superintendent returned he was quite surprised because I think he wanted it to be his idea. He was rather pleased though.'

Under the triumvirate of Mr Greene, Matron Belle Britain and Dr Francis Pilkington, Medical Superintendent, Moorhaven Hospital began to gain national recognition. Mr Greene encouraged general nurses to gain experience in psychiatric nursing. The King's Fund also began to send their matrons and administrators there on placements. Mr Greene was now a regular lecturer at the King's Fund, and he was appointed to the Salmon Committee on the reorganization of nursing management, working closely with Muriel Powell, Matron of St George's Hospital, London. Mr Greene was the first man to be awarded a British Commonwealth Nurses' War Memorial Fund scholarship.

I was interviewed by a panel that included Countess Mountbatten. One of these scholarships was the Countess Mountbatten scholarship – she insisted that I have it as she remembered me from Colombo. With this I travelled to the Scandinavian countries to study their highly regarded hospital systems. I was fortunate enough to be able to take my family with me, including the children. They had to keep detailed records for their school in England.

John Greene proved to be a powerful catalyst for change and he worked tirelessly to improve the status of mental health nursing. The NHS Retirement Fellowship was conceived at a party gathering at the Greenes' house, when guests including Elise Gordon and Muriel Powell discussed the concept. The launch was held at the Queen's Hotel in Cheltenham, and from there the Fellowship spread throughout the country. Hospitals were soon to move towards single senior appointments. Mr Greene applied for, and was appointed to, the post of Chief Nurse of Cornwall from 1969-74. Now responsible for general hospitals as well as mental health hospitals, he was to implement the Salmon Structure. As did many other people, Greene thought it was good in parts, but not altogether. He did, however, see the value in giving nurses a stronger voice. From 1974 to 1978 he was Area Nursing Officer for Gloucestershire.

A Chief Male Nurses' Association was formed by a group of senior male staff who got together to enact change. Mr Greene became President. This association then amalgamated with the Matrons of the Mental Hospitals, and Matrons of the Mental Handicap Hospitals. Following this, the Matrons of the General Hospitals (the Association of Hospital Matrons) invited them to merge further into a Chief and Principal Nurses' Association. Inheriting the chain of office, Mr Greene was appointed the first male President.

> In this role I felt that one of my main achievements was to lead the psychiatric nursing service away from its unfortunate low status, and bring it [amongst] much respected and admired services. As President of the association, I felt I was representing this advancement.

Before his retirement, Mr Greene spent time on hospital inspections and educational boards. He gained the OBE in 1973 for outstanding services to the hospital and nursing profession.

Through the work of nurse leaders, the psychiatric nursing services have advanced beyond all recognition. Psychiatric nursing is now a modern, progressive service, integrated into the mainstream of health provision. The old ways of nursing the poor have become nursing history. The workhouse infirmaries that Miss Pringle and Miss Barker made such a difference to continued to exist even as late as the 1940s, but they were then taken over by the new National Health Service.

These workhouses were vile places. Having taken over the work of the monasteries, they drew a crowd of unsavoury and uneducated staff. The poor, kept as virtual prisoners within them, suffered cruelty and neglect beyond imagination. With guardians who believed that pauperism was a sickness to be remedied by hard work, conditions could be harsh. There were as many as seventy thousand homeless people before the First World War, and thirty thousand prior to the Second World War, who relied totally on these institutions for shelter and medical care. In the early 1900s there were over a hundred thousand inmates of these workhouses. Before 1948 these institutions had separate 'casual' wards run by the Master and Matron, often housing sixty vagrants at a time. On the first day of each month, every casual ward occupant was medically examined, and if it was found necessary for that particular person to be admitted, Matron was required to provide a bed immediately.

By the time Lionel and Beryl Lewis came to be Master and Matron, the idea that being a pauper was some sort of disease had been largely consigned to the history books. Although pauperism remained feared by the general population, prejudices against it were being broken down due to the persistent efforts of people like Mr and Mrs Lewis. In workhouse infirmaries, there was an interchange between the sick in the workhouse and the sick in hospital, with the infirmary hospital still divided into male and female sections. All conditions were nursed, both surgical and medical. In the larger institutions they also included maternity and children's wards. Matron was firmly in charge.

Mr Lewis began workhouse life as a Junior Clerk at Newport, Monmouthshire in 1930. The institution accommodated over five hundred residents, in contrast to cities like Liverpool, Manchester and Sheffield where over two thousand were housed. Matron Rosa Slack had responsibility for the whole institution, and Miss Thom assisted her as Superintendent of Nurses.

At Newport there was a separate 'Labour' Master and Mistress. They were directly accountable to the Master and Matron, and were responsible for setting the casual ward inmates to work and making sure that they were fed properly.

They were also charged with checking that the 'casuals' received regular physical examinations.

The institutions operated under their own set of regulations A good knowledge of these proved essential to succeed in the interview when Mr Lewis applied for the post of Assistant Master at Green Lane Institution, Manchester.

For my interview I was put in front of a panel of about fifty members of the board of governors, and this was only for the post of Assistant Master. The first thing they did was to give me a list of public assistance questions. They immediately asked, 'What do you know about Section 22?' To gain time while I read it I said, 'Not much'. Fortunately the board found this funny. By the time they had settled again I had read and understood the question. It was to do with punishment of lunatics in mental wards. The whole interview was about the orders. It was important to them because they were running the establishment based on these.

Having survived the selection process, Mr Lewis found that the rules applied just as strictly to himself. He had to be available for duty the whole time except on Monday, Wednesday and Friday evenings when he could go out from six until ten o'clock at night. Not only that, he was also on call most nights.

I was often called in the middle of the night if a lunatic was going berserk to authorize their being put into a padded cell. It could only be done on my signature, ratified by the Medical Officer the next day. Sometimes I could be called three times in a night. If I had a night with only one case I thought it was absolutely marvellous.

The hospital was on three storeys within the precincts of the grounds, but separate from the main workhouse. Miss Price, under Matron Ryder and George Edgar Ryder, the Master, supervised the infirmary. Miss Price, Superintendent of Nurses, took charge of the daily running of the infirmary, but she remained responsible to the Master and Matron for all her requirements. She was also responsible for hygiene and for the behaviour of all female staff.

> Matron Ryder was a rather overpowering character, kept everyone on their toes, but she was fair. She was undoubtedly quite dominating and domineering in her handling of the staff. She was a well-built lady with quite an air of authority. [That is] probably why we did not have any nursing staff problems. Even though they were undoubtedly in fear and trembling when she did her rounds, and especially at inventory times, it was a very happy place nevertheless.

Moving on to a workhouse in Kingston, Mr Lewis witnessed the results of local policy decisions regarding mental ill health. Whereas Monmouthshire had about two hundred 'lunatic' cases residing within the workhouse infirmary, Kingston had none. Different counties had different policies for absorbing these people, and such was the pressure on mental hospitals that they were able to help only in the most severe of cases.

The following list is representative of the duties of an infirmary matron at the end of the nineteenth century. The first three articles (of twelve) place the matron clearly at the head of nursing within these institutions:

- To superintend the whole of the nursing staff and nursing arrangements of the Infirmary, subject in all matters to the approval of the Medical Superintendent.
- To aid the Medical Superintendent, and in his absence the Assistant to the Medical Superintendent, in enforcing order, punctuality, cleanliness, and the due observation of all regulations for the government of the Infirmary (including the Nurses' Home) on the part of the female servants therein, and to report to the Committee any negligence or other misconduct on the part of such female servants which may come to her knowledge.
- To cause the paupers, upon their admission, to be cleansed and to be properly clothed and placed in their proper wards,

unless the Medical Superintendent objects, or gives any special direction in the care.

- To hold, once a fortnight during the months of October to April (inclusive), a class for the practice of all kinds of bandaging and instruction in the principles of nursing, and to give instruction to the Nurses and Probationers in bedside nursing in different wards, and to keep a record of all such instruction and the Nurses' attendance thereat.
- To keep a Report Book, in which she shall report to the Infirmary Committee, through the Medical Superintendent, at each of the Meetings.

In 1932 Miss Beryl Jarrett, the future Mrs Lewis, started her training at St Woolos Hospital, Newport, Monmouthshire, gaining her SRN in 1935. After a year of midwifery training at the Royal Infirmary, Bristol, she returned to St Woolos Hospital as a staff nurse and was quickly promoted to Ward Sister, then Theatre Sister in 1938. A year later she became Night Sister, with responsibility for the whole hospital at night. Miss Jarrett was then appointed Senior Theatre Sister at Richmond Hospital, Surrey. When Mr Lewis was at the Central Relief Institution, Kingston upon Thames, they could spend more time together. They used to meet at six o'clock and be back for ten. Miss Jarrett gained excellent reports throughout both her student and midwifery training, showing what a dedicated and hard-working nurse she was. From this good start, and her determination to get on in the nursing profession, Miss Jarrett would be successful, and would gain a high position in any branch of nursing. Her choice was that she would have both a career and a marriage.

The war broke out and Lionel and Beryl decided that before he got called up, they should marry. They started to apply for joint appointments, and the one they chose was Master and Matron of St James Hospital (The Institution), Gravesend. The establishment had a hundred and ninety-eight beds and was half hospital and half home cases or vagrants. Having secured a married couple's posting while they were still single people, they had to marry rather more quickly than they had anticipated. Mr Lewis recalls:

> We had to marry in a hurry. You could not get away with cohabiting then. I suppose it was a sort of shotgun wedding. We were married at the church on the top of Richmond Hill. So we began our married lives as Master and Matron – I never did know who was the real boss!

The positions of Master and Matron were reserved exclusively for married couples. It was very demanding and meant running both a household and a business at the same time. This was more due to tradition than any practical arrangement, the idea being that a couple would bring a more 'homely' atmosphere to the institution. There were some separate appointments, but they were unusual.

On arrival at St James Hospital, Mr and Mrs Lewis found themselves in a rather peculiar situation. Unusually, there were a temporary Master and Matron running the institution. Mr Lewis found the handover of authority very straightforward, but Mrs Lewis experienced political resistance – the temporary Matron, who was from Dartford Hospital, had been instructed by the Chairman of the Workhouse Committee to continue supervising the hospital, so in effect both matrons were now in charge. Mrs Lewis could not assume the duties of Matron until the situation was resolved, but the chairman of the committee insisted that the arrangement should carry on. He insisted that 'even on a ship you have a captain and a first mate', which implied that he regarded the Matron of Dartford as the Captain, and Mrs Lewis as the First Mate. Refusing to accept this arrangement, Mr and Mrs Lewis took the case to Maidstone County Hall for arbitration. The court proclaimed the situation unacceptable, and Mrs Lewis won her rightful status as Matron of the hospital.

Not long after their arrival, a major incident nearly ended the newly weds' lives. The war was at its height in December 1940, and German bombers were busy attacking the Gravesend area.

Every night we had fire-watchers out because of the Blitz. We ended up sleeping in the big committee room where there was a sort of strong room; we could push in a single bed and manage to get a few hours' sleep. We were in bed and about twenty feet outside was a big lawn, where a thousand-pound bomb dropped. Fortunately there had been a lot of rain so the ground was very soft. It buried deep into the earth so the explosion went upwards rather than outwards. The building we were in was badly damaged but we were OK. Naturally when the staff came out to see what had happened, they expected to find us killed but apart from the shock and noise, we survived.

A reception centre was set up at St James Hospital for abandoned, abused and orphaned children. Mrs Lewis was Matron. There they received children, cleaned them and prepared them before they went to children's homes in the country. Mr and Mrs Lewis were very committed to the children, and would go with them when they were moved to the home.

One of the worst examples we saw were two children of about three or four who had been found sleeping in mattresses in a house in Gravesend. They had slit the mattresses with all the grey flock inside and slept in there. Their heads were absolutely covered in lice and they had maggot-infested sores. We cleaned them up and took them to the children's home nearby. The parents were sentenced to six months' imprisonment.

In 1945, Mr and Mrs Lewis were informed that there was a vacancy in Faversham. They went down by train, as there was no petrol at the time. 'The taxi was waiting at the station, and when we got to the hospital the driver said, "Are you the new master and matron of Bensted House?" We said, "Not yet", and he said, "God help you if you do take it, everybody is related to everybody else." We thought, well that's a good start. Nevertheless we took the job.'

By now, infirmary matrons' duties were more tied in with supervising the nurses:

1. Supervise the whole of the nursing staff and the nursing arrangements, including the training of probationers;
2. Superintend the female servants and domestic arrangements, and aid the Medical Superintendent in enforcing order, punctuality and the observance of all rules made for the guidance of such staff;
3. Take charge of, and cause to be kept in proper condition, all instruments and appliances in the wards, and all crockery, cooking utensils, and other domestic appliances when issued for use in the wards, and from time to time to check the accuracy of the requisitions sent in from the wards.[2]

One of the first things Matron Lewis had to do was turn round traditional 'custom and practice' within the hospital. These were routines that staff had become accustomed to for many years. She insisted on a set of basic principles; these included respect for privacy, acknowledgement of dignity, and avoidance of restraint measures. It was not unusual for wandering patients to be tied to their chairs by wrapping sheets round their waists and tying these to the backs of the chair. Regular meetings with the Sister and staff of each ward, and with the medical officer, helped to ensure compliance.

Matron Lewis's duties also included the ordering and dispensing of all medicines, dealing with correspondence, and the ward rounds. Each day she made a point of seeing and speaking to all the patients and staff, but like other matrons, Mrs Lewis was more than just the Hospital Matron; she was equally concerned about the welfare of patients' relatives, acutely aware of the pressure that illness brings to a family. She also kept a watchful and benevolent eye on her staff so that difficulties could be attended to promptly.

NHS restructuring resulted in St James Hospital being taken over in 1948 by the Canterbury Group. Mrs Lewis accepted the changes this meant. She still kept the important contact with patients which she so enjoyed, despite attending the Regional Hospital Board and other committee meetings. Throughout her career it was this direct communication with patients that had given her the most pleasure. What did become apparent after the restructuring were the changes in authority.

It was the Group system that defused authority. We used to be able to transfer patients within our own institution; now there was an admissions person appointed to deal with admissions. The dispensary system changed as dispensing was all done at Canterbury. You suddenly had a Group Engineer, a Group Domestic Supervisor, and Group Laundry and Finance Departments all wanting to justify their existence. Did we gain anything from this? Look at today, nobody is accountable any more!

There were Regional Hospital Boards (RHB) and these were divided into Groups. Some institutions ended up being administered by the County Council and others by Regional Hospital Boards. The situation was a nightmare of bureaucracy. It was possible to have the County Council charging the RHB for looking after the hospital patients, and the RHB charging the County Council for looking after the elderly, 'A proper mess-up.' Increases in administration took the focus away from patient care. This proved to be a change too far for Mrs Lewis, who retired from nursing after thirty-six years in 1968.

Mr Lewis realized that the job was changing faster than he was when he was told he had to join a group of managers to talk out their personal problems. The idea was that by doing this they could understand the problems of others.

You had to throw your personal problems into the circle and believe me you had to have a problem! On one occasion, I turned to Mary and said, 'How are you, Mary? It is a lovely day today, isn't it?' There had been silence up till then, so they immediately picked on me and said, 'Lionel, why did you say that?' With that I was then almost thrown into the middle of the circle. It was all getting a bit of a nonsense really, so I thought, this is the time to go.

Mr Lewis had forty-nine years of service behind him. He was the National President of the Association of Hospital and Welfare Administrators (formerly Masters and Matrons) from 1958–59, and became a National Life Honorary Member.

Betty Connor was also destined for the role of matron. She lived with her parents at the 'Old Lodge' which was built, along with the Bolton Workhouse (Fishpool), in 1860. The house was situated at the main gates by the institution. Its original purpose was to accommodate the admission of prospective inmates. The resident Porter and Portress saw that the inmates were bathed, de-loused if necessary, then dressed in 'uniforms'. Inmates were then placed in appropriate accommodation within the main building, in other words the elderly, younger homeless, and sick people went to the hospital, and the 'mental' patients to a secure building.

As a little three-year-old girl, I waited with my mother and father outside the big iron gates of the institution. Soon a porter opened the gates and let us in to go along the drive to a mass of dark buildings. Although I did not know it then, this was to be my home for more than twenty years. I lived there not as an inmate, but because I was the daughter of the resident Engineer.[3]

I have vivid memories of going into the day rooms and talking to the inmates and, more importantly, listening as the people were so glad to have someone to talk to. Here I think I learned how to approach older people and the mentally ill. I particularly remember Christmas, and on Boxing Day the inmates had their special Christmas Dinner with a visit from the 'Board of Guardians'. Staff always gave a concert in the evening, and the Master and Matron would really let their hair down.

Mr and Mrs Burns were the Master and Matron when Betty Connor arrived. Mr and Mrs Don Ernsting were then the

Master and Matron from 1946-1964 and saw in many notable changes, not least the National Health Service reorganization in 1948. Mr and Mrs Ernsting had previously been Master and Matron of the Woodbine House Public Assistance Institution and Emergency Medical Services Hospital from 1939-45. The hospital had been used extensively during the war; all of Matron Ernsting's nursing skills had been needed. One thousand servicemen were treated as inpatients each year, in addition to hundreds of civilians. One notable change that occurred during the Ernstings' time was the introduction of spectacles for residents; out of 450 residents, as many as 173 benefited. Matron Ernsting also inaugurated 'diversional' therapy, the forerunner to occupational therapy, for residents in all the wards, including the mental wards. In 1949 Mr Ernsting assumed the duties of Deputy Group Secretary of Bolton and District Hospital.

Mrs Connor had always been interested in nursing and was reading the *Nursing Mirror* as a young girl. She also had first-hand experience of being admitted to hospitals, so could understand a patient's perspective. During one of her stays in hospital, the doctor asked her why she was reading a nursing magazine. When she replied that she wanted to be a nurse, he said sternly, 'Nursing isn't all uniform and starch, you know!' It seems that her confidence unsettled him. When she left her convent school at seventeen to start her nursing career, one of the nuns said, 'Do you think that you are strong enough to be a nurse?' Fortunately, neither of these episodes put her off nursing.

Wrightington Hospital near Wigan is now a centre of excellence for orthopaedic surgery, but when Mrs Connor started nursing in 1941, it was an isolation hospital for tuberculosis.

On arrival, and without any ceremony, I was given my uniform, shown how to pleat up my cap, and taken to Matron's Office. From there I was immediately placed on a ward. The orthopaedic wards were hard work as the patients were on heavy steel frames and had to be 'turned' for bedbaths and pressure area treatment. The junior nurses had to push the beds out onto the veranda in the morning and back in again for teatime. We had to learn how to sweep and clean a ward.

At eighteen Mrs Connor commenced her nurse training at Townley Hospital (formerly Fishpool Institution), Bolton. Matron Bethel firmly told her that she had to live in the nurses' accommodation, even though her own home was in the grounds of the hospital. The nurses' home had no central heating, but apart from that it became a home from home. As her father was the hospital engineer, he used to be called out to see to any repairs. He would be furious when he found the fires turned upside down to heat food on.

> Matron Bethel was very stately and could be very strict. She once caught me in the kitchen drinking tea, but all she said was 'No saucer, nurse?' One of the Sisters made us drink Marmite made with hot milk 'Drink it, nurse, it will do you good!'

Miss Rushton married William Connor in 1950 and, as a couple, they could now apply for joint positions. With Mrs Connor's nursing skills and Mr Connor's administration skills, they were appointed as Assistant Superintendent and Assistant Matron at Hillborough, a large institution in Worcester, in 1957. This was to be the stepping stone to managing their own institution. Late in 1958, they were appointed Superintendent and Matron at East View, Stow-on-the-Wold in Gloucester. East View was known as a 'joint user', with both ambulant and chronically sick patients. This meant that the Connors were responsible to both the Banbury District Hospital Management Committee and Gloucester County Council Welfare Department.

> In a way the 'joint user' was a good idea for some purposes; however we had two 'bosses', which sometimes created difficulties. This type of care is now a thing of the past in the public sector. We had very little time off-duty and high levels of responsibility. This meant juggling the needs of the matron role with the responsibilities of bringing up two children who

used to love to talk to the residents, as I had as a child in Bolton. Unfortunately for us it did not work.

After a break of a few years they later obtained a joint appointment as Officer in Charge and Matron of a residential home with Salford Social Services, where they remained until retirement.

The amazing leadership and contribution these men and women provided over the years cannot be stated too highly. Nursing the 'mentally deficient' and the elderly, and care of the dying had for years been the unpopular end of nursing, and were for many years shunned by nurses who considered this sort of work to be second rate. Many of these sectors of nursing now have nurse specialists in both hospitals and the community, and all are making great advances in medical and nursing care.

Notes

1. Greene, J., *Dominic Remembers, Life in County Clare 1916 to 1935.* (K. Greene, Newcastle upon Tyne, 1994)
2. Jennings, W.I., *The Poor Law Code* (Charles Knight & Co. Ltd., London, circa 1930)
3. Connor, B., *A Pauper Palace: A History of Fishpool Institution* (N. Richardson, Bolton, 1989)

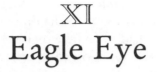

XI
Eagle Eye

The matron job was a phenomenon and the embodiment of ingrained principles. Like a diamond, Matron had many facets that left a lasting impression. The memories nurses have of her are enduring, indicative of the high level of emotion associated with her. Describing her with a mixture of awe and fear, nurse contributors show their ultimate respect for matron, bringing the past to life and revealing matron in all her glory. Matron was the dominant figure in the hospital, rigorously upholding the very high standards of a self-assured and dignified profession.

Infections were, and still are, a major cause of illness and death in hospitals. Prior to the development of penicillin in 1941, the only way to prevent cross-infection was by scrupulous cleanliness, carefully supervised by the matron. Matron, as head of nursing care, was the key figure in the fight against infection, and cleanliness was her primary weapon. Matron's activities are often viewed as overly obsessive. Her emphasis was on the tidiness of linen rooms, neatness of dress and cleanliness of wards, also on nurses' deportment, attitudes and habits. They were the matron's own eccentricities, but these standards brought nursing out of the dark ages and turned it into a much respected profession. These standards were readily accepted by nurses and adhering to them was a sign that one took pride in one's work.

Muriel Handley, a nurse at the former Wolverhampton Royal Hospital, remembers matron's activities as having a direct bearing on infection control. Everything had a purpose;

cleanliness and neatness were never a waste of time as they were the only barriers they had against cross-infection. There were no antibiotics at that time. The reason why nurses did all the cleaning was because it was in the patients' interest to do it: prevention of cross-infection was vital. In Muriel's day, nurses took off aprons to go to the dining room, and if they changed ward, they had to change their whole uniform. 'That is why relatives were not allowed to sit on beds!' Before the Second World War, and for some time after, all soiled linen was rinsed and counted before being put in the laundry baskets. Bedpans made of porcelain or enamel were thoroughly cleansed, washed and sterilized, and the nursing staff made up their own bottles of disinfectant such as carbolic.

Visiting hours were busy times for nurses. During this period they would leave their patients in the company of relatives and get on with other work. The nurses made up individual dressings and packed them in metal drums ready for the autoclave (sterilizer). The ward autoclave would need emptying, and the ward sisters would often clean it with Brasso until it shone. All the sputum mugs, urine bottles and bedpans had to be neatly lined up. The ward number would be sewn on to new linen by nurses, and this was checked by matron at the monthly ward inventory. Trolleys and trays were set out for special treatments. All equipment had to be boiled both before and after use. Neatness and orderliness were so important, from making a bed to personal tidiness. It was not just an image, it was the nursing standard that the matron demanded at that time. It was a form of discipline that had been handed down from the earlier army and religious orders, but the nurses accepted it; it was not a bind, they were proud to be smart and clean, and saw its importance. To see that her nurses were meeting the standards required, matron or her deputies would do daily rounds of the hospital. Depending on the size of the hospital, rounds could be weekly, or twice daily. Of all matron's activities, it had to be the ward round that generated their fearsome reputation as dragons or battle-axes.

Cliff Morgan, as a student nurse, describes matron as a

proud and honourable presence. A woman of five-foot two, 'she would enter the ward like a seven-foot stately galleon'. Matron equally affected Ken Standing, a patient in a military hospital during the 1950s. He recalls the special atmosphere created the moment matron would enter the ward. When the Surgeon Commander came onto the ward for his round, the men would always be very respectful; they would extinguish their cigarettes, clear away magazines, turn the radios down and talk quietly, but when Matron entered the ward it was very different. Despite being of a lower rank, she had the greater air of authority. Ken Standing points out how remarkable it all was: they would find themselves sitting to attention beside their beds, or lying to attention in beds with the sheets tightly pulled up to their necks. The place would be in silence, the hard-nosed sailors would not say a word. 'We respected her you see.'

Emily Soper (née Dick) started her training at Stobhill General Hospital, Glasgow, in 1938. Some wards of the hospital have more recently been used to film the the television programme 'Cardiac Arrest', which Emily finds amusing to watch. She feels that her old matron must be turning in her grave at the turn of events. Emily explained how matron's uniform was an image of confidence and competence. On duty the uniform had to be immaculate. They wore a long-sleeved button-up frock of a bluish denim cloth. When the sleeves were rolled up, they wore frilled cotton over-sleeves with hard button cuffs. The collar was also of a hard starched material. All this was topped by a starched white apron and hard, white belt around the middle. Nurses' caps were also starched, made of white cotton with a drawstring, and had to be pleated neatly. Some of the nurses did have an artistic touch, their caps were virtually works of art. They could not wear this uniform outside the hospital. 'I am sure the uniforms worn today do not command [as much] respect as the old traditional style; and the patients knew who was who!'

Emily Soper also remembers Matron with awe. She was a tall, sturdy Highlander, a strict disciplinarian with equally powerful deputies by her side. When the infamous 'bush tele-

graph' informed the ward that matron was on her way, everyone from Sister to the most junior nurse would be poised and
tense. She would sweep into the ward like a 'battleship', missing nothing, not even the jugs of water. If the jugs were not
filled to a certain level, she would tell the nurse to fill them
and not move until it was done. Withered flowers were not
tolerated, and no patient would dare cross their legs in bed.
Not only was Matron scanning the patients, she was also
inspecting each member of staff. They were all being scrutinized just as carefully! If a nurse's cap was askew or not
pleated perfectly, that nurse was to report to Matron's office
the next morning; any signs of a ladder in their black stockings and the punishment was the same. 'Even the doctors were
terrified of her. You might, perhaps, see a young one cringing
in a dark corner of the ward when this Amazon of a woman
approached. She saw every one of them, but usually ignored
their presence for, to her, they were quite insignificant; they
were not her nurses!'

Josephine Chadkirk completed her training at a small
general hospital near Hebburn. Her matron was of the 'old
type', strict but fair, with exacting standards. Everything had
to be ready for matron's ward round and woe betide anyone
who hadn't finished their task, or at least tried to make it look
as though they had. Everything was cleared away, ambulant
patients were seated in a chair beside their bed, at a specific
angle and distance from the bed (otherwise they were trussed
up in bed so that they could not move, looking for all the
world as though their bodies ended where the bed covers
began). After a few months, nurses developed a sixth sense as
to who was advancing towards the ward door and when.

Monica Matterson, (née Johnson) trained at Scarborough
General Hospital in 1943, where Miss Ann Escolme was
matron. Miss Escolme was described by Monica as a 'very
genteel lady'. She still remembers the ward round well, noting
how matron inspected her domain in three phases: first the
environment, then the patients, and finally her nurses.
Cleaning of the ward had to be done before matron appeared.
There would be a frenzy of sweeping, dusting, and tidying

of lockers. Bedpans were cleaned and neatly lined up on the shelf, and the sluice room would be left spotless and orderly. In the sluice room was a white porcelain gully with a brass trap with all the mess in it, and matron would always inspect that. The draining boards were made of teak and were polished until they shone. Matron inspected every toilet and every part of the kitchen. Beds were lined up with the sheets turned back to the distance between elbow and fingertip. When matron had inspected all this she would then start with the patients. She would speak to all of them, but only spoke to the nurse if there was something she didn't approve of. 'Matron Escolme never raised her voice, she always spoke nicely. I am sure the ward maids were revered more than we were, because second to the patients, cleanliness was more important than any other consideration.'

Chris Farmer (née McCrea) trained at Ballochmyle Hospital, an emergency military services hospital (EMS) in Scotland, in 1945. The bed occupancy was over one thousand people. To an eighteen-year-old, Matron Gillanders was a very imposing person. She was a smart lady, always looking magnificent in her uniform with her large white cap tied under her chin. 'I never saw her in anything else but her uniform. She was always impeccable.' When matron entered the ward it was enough to scare the life out of them. There was a deathly hush, the doors would be flung open and in would march matron. She would first sweep into the Sisters' office. After this, she would proceed down the ward, eyeing everything. It seemed that she missed nothing. Matron was a terrifying sight to Chris and the other students. 'Yet there was never anything to be frightened of, it was her aura, the image, that was so frightening; a small lady, she had an immense presence.' Sister would have them all hyped up anyway. Was their hair right? Pull your sleeves down! Put your cuffs on properly! Attention to detail was, of course, matron's forte. Some of the standards insisted upon can seem rather extreme, for example the ward layout, which was a work of art.

At some hospitals, a board was used to do the lining up of the beds. It was laid on the floor to a line running down the length of the ward and the beds had to be pushed exactly to the edge, with the wheels exactly pointing at each other so that no one would trip over them; it made sense then. Billie Godfrey (née Bailey) trained at St Charles Hospital, London, under Matron Miss Gibb, and reflected on the precision with which wards were arranged. The beds had to be lined up inch-perfect; she had even seen it done with a piece of string. All the pillows had to be in line, with the tucked in part pointing in the opposite direction to the ward entrance. Even the patients were affected by the 'matron effect', not so much by trying to please her as trying not to draw attention to themselves. They would comb their hair, check that there were no creases in their sheets, ensure that they looked their very best, see that there were no newspapers visible and that their lockers were tidy. Gladys Tubb trained at Peterborough Memorial Hospital, where Miss Naismith was Matron. She had a reputation for having very sharp eyes; Matron missed nothing. Most days she would just appear from seemingly nowhere, but every Sunday she would have a thorough inspection of the wards. On the medical wards they used lots of kaolin poultices. It didn't need to be sterile and because they were so short of staff, someone would make up a very large poultice and keep it hot on top of the sterilizer. The nurses would then cut pieces off, as and when needed. One day matron appeared, picked up the poultice by one corner, and deposited the lot in the pedal bin. 'Boy, did we get a ticking off! But I cannot talk too highly of her, she was a wonderful matron and so good to us student nurses.'

Sheila Simmons will never forget acting up for Sister at a London teaching hospital in 1938. 'On my first day of acting up in the absence of the ward sister, it was matron's round. She had just had three days off and was not entirely conversant with the new patients.' On entering the ward, Matron and the assistant matron (nicknamed 'Miss Echo') stood examining the line of beds. Matron immediately marched to the third bed and summoned nurse Simmons. The nurse quaked; was Matron going to ask her the diagnosis and treatment? (In those days there was no excuse for not knowing.) To her initial relief she told her that Mr N— had been operated on three days previously for a perforated duodenum. 'But then, "Legs" Matron announced to the world, "Mr N's legs are crossed. Nurse, see that they are uncrossed now and that they are not crossed again." ' Never to be outdone, the assistant matron whispered not too quietly behind her, 'Crossed legs are important, nurse.' Matron always talked directly to the patient, but when any sort of misdemeanour occurred, such as 'legs', the culprit was made painfully aware. The procession continued without further mishaps until the round was completed. 'On leaving, Matron again reminded me about the importance of legs; this time with a short, not unfriendly lecture on the perils of thrombosis. With that she looked down the ward one last time and said, "Good order, Sister." Yip, I thought. She called me Sister.'

As a patient, Captain Julia Simpson RN had first-hand experience of the instant panic amongst the nurses that an imminent ward round caused. She was on an officers' training course when she was admitted as a patient to the Herbert Military Hospital, Woolwich. Having been there a while, Captain Simpson was becoming a little fed up, so one of the nurses suggested that she do her hair and lighten it a little with bleach. They were in the bathroom with the bleach on Captain Simpson's hair when one of the nurses rushed in and said that Matron was on the ward! That was it! At once the nurses gathered all the equipment together and shot off, leaving Captain Simpson with dripping hair. 'It was some time before the nurse returned and by then my brown hair was blonde.'

Matron knew all the patients. It never failed to amaze nurses how Matron could remember so many patients' names and their treatments, but this reflected the belief that one couldn't care for a patient if one did not know them, their name and what was wrong with them; otherwise they would be just anonymous bodies in beds. To some extent this knowledge was facilitated by patients remaining in hospital for much longer periods of time. For example, in those days someone with a heart condition could be in hospital for up to ten weeks, and an appendicectomy patient might stay for seven to ten days. The emphasis on nursing was the provision of good basic care, and good basic care was given. The source of matron's knowledge was a strong team of assistant matrons who supported her. They collected written reports from every ward for matron's attention, and she studied them carefully.

Vera Payne, a teaching hospital nurse, found the ward round an excellent learning experience even though she dreaded it. It forced the kind of attention to detail that nursing had become renowned for. As part of matron's round, the nurses would be quizzed on the name of every patient, their diagnosis, their condition, and their treatment. It could be a terrifying experience, and many nurses went through it. Vera remembers one particular occasion when the assistant matron asked her how much blood loss a patient had suffered during the operation. 'I could not figure out how she could have had the information. Luckily, I did know and did not make it up, otherwise I would have been in trouble.'

Jean, a nurse at Peterborough Hospital, accompanied matron on her ward round. A junior nurse at the time, she was nevertheless expected to know the name of every patient. She struggled on the very last patient, who had been admitted the night before for an emergency appendix operation. She did not know the name of the patient and, feeling very stressed by now, in sheer desperation said, 'This is last night's appendix.' Immediately she shrank under matron's gaze. 'Nurse, this is not an appendix, but a patient who has had an appendicectomy. Find out his name and apologize to him now!'

Tom Diamond trained at Guy's Hospital, London. He remembers his experiences of knowing patients. At Guy's Hospital, the ward round could be terrifying. Matron knew all the patients, therefore, as a student or staff nurse, he felt he had to as well.. Matron or one of her assistants would come to the ward door and pick on a student, not the ward sister. They would start at the first bed and proceed round to the last one, and matron would expect to be told who each person was, the diagnosis, their date of birth, if they were married, if they were in the services, if they were recovering, and when were they going home. This was done for all twenty-five beds without fail. Students had to remember the ones they already knew and also the new ones, as they did not want to be caught out. It was easier by the time Tom started because the patients had boards at the bottom of the beds, so a lot of the information was already there, but before this nurses had to do the same thing purely from memory. If the nurse did not know, she had to say so, because the matron certainly knew. 'How did they know? Because they did it every day of their lives! I'll tell you, if you got anything wrong you really knew about it. You got a strong message from the assistant matron, then you got it in the neck from Sister, and you only let her down once.' Tom, however, thinks the nurses built that fear up themselves. He does not remember a single incident in the whole of his training where he could say matron was unfair or gave him cause to be frightened of her. 'I think it was a culture that was built up amongst us all – you know, "Oh! It's Matron coming, jump to it!" " You have to go to see Matron, so you must be in trouble!" '

Not knowing the patient was one thing, but not knowing the name of equipment was quite another. Josephine Chadkirk found out how important the correct identification of equipment was to matron, and how long her memory could be. One day Josephine was rushing along the corridor when matron asked her what she was carrying. 'A sphygmo, Matron.' 'A what, student nurse?' 'A sphygmo.' 'Now tell me the correct name.' 'A sphygmo . . . mame . . . ter, Matron.' She was held up for quite a while being made to get her tongue around the word 'sphygmomanometer', and having to spell it correctly. Then Josephine had to explain to an irate doctor and ward sister why it had taken her so long to go to the ward next door. For the next couple of years whenever matron saw her, she would say with her wonderful smile, 'Well, student nurse?', and Josephine would go through the routine of spelling it again.

In Matron's day, hospitals were funded by voluntary donations, so it was Matron's role to ensure that these gifts were not abused, and that costs were kept to a minimum and losses reduced. Despite the logic behind them, ward inventories were fearful experiences for the staff. Each item had to gleam and be available for matron and her assistant matrons to view. They counted every single item on the ward; the linen room, sluice room and the kitchen were checked against the ward inventory. Everything had to be accounted for, every wheelchair, walking stick and bed-table. Matron was responsible for supplies on her wards and, with the charitable nature of hospital finance, she could be uncompromising about breakages'.

Most nurses working in hospitals prior to 1950 remember having to report to Matron's office if they broke equipment. Unfortunately for them, the humble thermometer proved to be the bane of their lives. This simple, but extraordinarily useful, piece of equipment was rather frail. To get the mercury down to the bottom of the thermometer, it was held with two fingers and given a quick flick of the wrist, However, nothing could have been easier than launching it under the bed, over to the next bed, or knocking it on something. The patients thought this was hilarious, and their own attempts ended with the same result. Gladys Tubb took the 'Walk of Despair', the route to matron's office, once when she went to report a breakage. She was on night duty, and when taking routine temperatures, broke a thermometer and found three other broken ones in a paste jar. Finding another two, she decided to take them all to Matron. Carrying the broken thermometers in a kidney dish, she knocked on Matron's office door. Matron was dumbfounded: Gladys had not only owned up to breaking one, but had brought them all in. She did not reprimand her. 'The other nurses were waiting for a crying nurse to come into the dining room, and were equally dumbfounded when I was perfectly OK.'

For Billie Godfrey, a visit to matron's office turned out disastrously. It was the first time she had to see the matron with a broken thermometer, and the first time she had been to matron's office at all. Standing outside, waiting to be summoned, she remembers that she was visibly quaking. In her hand was the offending article, in a dish covered by a cloth. The bell sounded. Billie entered and was sternly asked what had happened. 'The patient broke it, Matron,' she bleated. 'Do not blame my patients, it is your responsibility, nurse. Be more careful in the future.' With that, matron turned to the cupboard behind her to pull out a drawer with the new thermometers in. The drawer stuck. She pulled again and the drawer shot right out, spilling thermometers all over the floor. Bits of broken thermometer were everywhere. Billie went to help matron, but was told in no uncertain terms to get out. Outside waiting, her friend had heard the racket and was by now equally scared. She had over-boiled a twenty-millilitre syringe. As Billie disappeared, nearly in tears, her friend timidly knocked on the door. With the syringe rattling in the metal kidney dish, she entered. Billie was waiting with a group of nurses, expecting the worst. Asked by her friends later what had happened, she said there had been quite a delay before she was called in, then when she entered and spluttered her apology for the ruined syringe, matron had held up her hand and said, 'Never mind, nurse. Accidents do happen!'

Roy Stallard was a student at Wolverhampton Royal Hospital where Miss Richie was matron. He remembers a colleague, a junior student, who was told to sterilize all the thermometers on the ward. Being eager to please, the student duly took all thirty-four of them to the sluice room and boiled them. It appears that the mechanism of temperature measurement had eluded him on that day. Causing great amusement throughout the hospital, somehow he survived his trip to matron's office.

Throughout matron's rule, high standards were achieved in infection control, aseptic techniques and bedside care. As a visible leader, matron kept up standards through ward rounds, and moral responsibility was maintained by those dreaded visits to matron's office. What a wonderful grounding and example it was to these young nurses! With her controls and checks, matron was shaping her nurses for the future, but she was not all 'discipline and starched aprons'. Although maintaining order was a significant part of her role, she was also responsible for the welfare of her staff. The young nurses in training were beginning their adult lives, and in matron's day girls were generally more inexperienced and immature than of the girls of today.

XII
Moral Guardian

At the time of the First World War, nurses still wore elaborate Victorian uniforms, said daily prayers, and paraded to church on Sundays. Hospital regulations also remained Victorian. By the end of the Second World War, however, attendance at church was voluntary, and although the values of duty and morality were still being upheld, they were being challenged by wider social changes. Nurse accommodation in many hospitals had changed very little, but ward sisters no longer lived on the wards.

Up until the late 1960s, matron's office dealt with everything to do with nursing; new appointments, dismissals, and changes in hospital regulations went through this office. There was no such thing as a personnel department; the majority of new recruits were young girls who immediately became the responsibility of the matron. These girls had been entrusted to matron by parents who expected their daughters to come to no harm whilst in her care in *in loco parentis*. Ann Parkin commenced training in 1942 and fully understood matron's problems. She thought that before the First World War, matron did not want any of her young ladies to be viewed by society as trollops. 'I got the tail end of it, the "must be in by ten o'clock". The nurses' home was known as the "nunnery" to the local lads in the town.'

Frances Trimmer points out the extreme naïvety of girls aged eighteen in the 1940s. When she entered training, the age of consent was twenty-one and the girls were very sexually unsophisticated. 'Just to show you how very naïve as young girls we were, we were so very puzzled when we found balloons in some of the soldiers' pockets.' As an eighteen-year-old in 1941, Elizabeth Bailey (née Downward) started her training at the Royal United Hospital in Bath. It was there where she was introduced to condoms, but for a more serious purpose. There was great confusion as to what should and should not be done where male patients were concerned. They used to shave the soldiers prior to theatre, but this was stopped and male orderlies were introduced. However, the nurses still had to continue to do these duties when there were no orderlies available. One thing she did have to get used to was using condoms, which she had never encountered before. Condoms were used to treat soldiers' injuries from land mines. When a soldier stepped on a mine, the blast went upwards doing dreadful damage to his penis and testicles. The condom was the only thing that would keep them together for healing. The nurses cut a hole in the end of the condom so the patient could go to the toilet. On the first occasion, Elizabeth did not have a clue what to do with the thing, so one of the orderlies said, 'Come here girl, I have got daughters of my own, I'll do it.' She soon learned, and had to withstand some ribbing, as her patients were only eighteen and nineteen years old themselves.

Under matron's rule, standards were exacting. Standards in society and in the nurses' own homes were more restrictive than today. Standards set in the school of nursing formed the basis of a nurse's education for life; initially, these were based on etiquette and deportment, but then they involved providing the best quality care in the clinical area.

In 1927, Lucy Baird (née Simon) commenced her first nursing experience at the Sunshine Home for Blind Babies in Birkdale, Lancashire. On her first day, she arrived in a Landau. The driver wore a uniform and a tall, black hat. It was the equivalent of the modern day taxi. One activity matron liked was for the nurses to attend church, which meant a three-mile walk into Southport. Lucy found the standards very strict. In their study books, the nurses had to write twenty-five times, 'When speaking to Matron or any superior person, we must stand with feet together and hands behind our backs.' Her daughter pointed out that after seventy-three years, her mother will still stand like this if she is waiting in a queue for something.

Emily Soper rather painfully remembers her own introduction to the setting of standards. She feels that the nurses were treated like children with everything so regimented. In the preliminary training school, weekdays were spent in the school, and two out of four weekends were spent in the wards. It was often a seven-day working week. 'I can remember making a mistake and [being] rapped over the knuckles with a ruler. Today I would be able to sue. It did us no harm though, no matter what they say now. It strengthened us, look what we came through.'

Elizabeth Bailey learned how the hierarchical system began even very low down the ladder. As a student, if a nurse wanted to say something to matron she never spoke to her directly. If there was anything to be said the senior nurse was told, she then told the staff nurse, who told the Sister, who in turn told the matron! It was exactly the same procedure with the consultant. When attending matron's office for whatever reason, if there was someone senior present, they stood back to let them go first. 'You really were much of the lower order then, but you also knew one day you would be staff nurse.'

Lynette King (née Brownhill) was a shy teenager, who had been to boarding school and had very little contact with the male species, when she entered hospital life. She would disappear and hide in the toilet at every opportunity. The ward sister would attempt to coax her out, but it was matron who thumped on the door, voice booming, ordering her to get on with the job. 'The patients are harmless, they would stand a much better chance of recovery if you were nursing them, and not hiding in the lavatory!' she shouted. She marched Lynette onto the ward and this somehow had the desired effect: her fear went, and she fell in love with the job. That particular ward became her favourite.

'Living in' was compulsory for trainee nurses, and entering the nurses' home was not too onerous for the majority, as most were used to restrictions at home anyway. They did have to get used to some strange practices though, such as beds being moved out of the rooms when male visitors arrived. For Monica Matterson, these living conditions in Yorkshire were quite harsh. The one thing she will never forget is that each day matron used to do a round of the nurses' home. If a nurse's bed wasn't made properly or if the room wasn't tidy, matron would strip the bed. Nurses were allowed only seven items on the dressing table and, if there were more, they would find them on the floor. Monica remembers her Nissen hut on the Yorkshire moors being so cold with only one radiator that the water would freeze in the bowl by the bedside. To keep warm, they borrowed long theatre socks and stone hot water bottles, but matron would 'raid' the bedrooms and take them back. 'You were really in trouble for that. It was not done individually, but as a group, so you ended up feeling terrible because she would put you down, sort of shame you . . .' For Gladys Tubb, coming from a large family, having her own room in a brick building was a blessing. The room consisted of an iron bed with a hard mattress, well-worn lino, a small rug, one plain chair, no bedside cupboard or lamp, no wardrobe, only a curtain across one corner with a few hooks below, a shelf for cases and a shelf for shoes. There was an old chest of drawers with a mirror, and an ancient wash-stand. There was no wash-basin in the room and nurses had to share the bathroom. What they did have was a radiator in every room, so it was usually warm. 'Coming from a large family and always having to share a bed, this was paradise. I had privacy at last!'

As a mature student (aged thirty), Betty Groves was allowed to live out much earlier than the other students, but matron was still very interested in her welfare. Betty had been home one morning and, walking over a railway bridge, got a piece of soot in her eye. She went to another hospital to get it cleaned and returned to duty in the afternoon. She said nothing because it did not seem appropriate, as it did not affect her ability to work. Matron sent for her and wanted to know if she was OK – she was genuinely concerned. 'I did not think to ask her how she had come by the information, but it was clear that even though I lived out, my welfare was still of concern to her.'

Juliette Diamond's life was still strictly monitored in the nurses' home when she started her training in 1960. They were even told how many socks, shoes and knickers to bring with them. The home sisters took the trainee nurses out the day after they started the job, to buy anything that they thought was missing from the list. This was all bought using the money the nurses took with them. 'They actually took us two by two down the road.' Being under the age of consent, the system was still very protective. The home sisters became the nurses' carers, and matron was like a Mother Superior. Despite the restrictions of 'living in', all the nurses agreed that in the nurses' home special bonds were formed, and friendships developed that lasted a lifetime. Letters of resignation would be written out on a regular basis, but they would be torn up after a cup of tea and a 'bellyache' with colleagues. There was also the fact that 'the more rules there were, the more fun it was breaking them.'

For nurses living in, meals were compulsory. It was matron's way of ensuring nurses ate a good meal, especially breakfast. Part of this was to ensure the nurses were not losing weight. Lunch was at midday, and nurses would be seated at long tables in order of seniority. Matron sat at the head of the sisters' table, and then the juniors, in descending rank. Grace was said before and after meals. At some hospitals the home sister would note if the nurses' appetites were normal, and also give out vitamin C and ferrous sulphate (iron) tablets.

Patricia Palmer, a student nurse in 1958 at Romsey Hospital, found herself responsible for putting mustard on the table on beef days. With only mustard powder available, it had to be made fresh. The nurses would sit and wait for the cook to bring in the roast, and if the way it was cooked did not suit matron, it would be sent back, although Patricia is sure that the same joint would be brought back to the table.

As the junior nurse, she was expected to ring the bell for the next course or dessert. To avoid keeping matron waiting, Patricia would only put a small helping of vegetables on her plate to avoid taking too long to eat. Consequently Patricia was invariably hungry.

Margaret Morris was eighteen when she started training at the Miller Voluntary Hospital, Greenwich, at the beginning of the Second World War. She would often go out in her uniform, along with her two friends, which was 'forbidden of course'. Seeing three nurses together in their uniforms 'and our lovely hats with bows tied under our chins', the London stall-holders would give them an apple or an extra piece of fruit. 'They did like to see us nurses, and for a real treat they would sometimes give us black silk stockings.' Back at the hospital, they knew they had to 'conform' at meal times. Monitoring the diet of nurses proved particularly important in the war. Their diet was often supplemented by sweets from patients. Chris Farmer lost weight because she was working in the operating theatre, not on the wards where she was used to being given sweets. The sweets had supplemented her diet to the extent that even matron noticed the weight loss.

For Sheila Clark and her nurse colleagues, chicken was not on the menu for Christmas during the war. Chicken at Christmas was a treat not often experienced for the rest of the year. The nurses had corned beef, cabbage and boiled potatoes, but the patients had the roast chicken. The following year, there was a vegetable patch just behind the nurses' home with the first crop of potatoes – matron believed in 'Digging for Victory' – the nurses decided to boil some new potatoes for themselves. They crept out and dug some up, but suddenly a voice called, 'Nurses, what are you doing?' It was matron. 'Put them back at once!' and she stood there while they did.

Mary Verrier volunteered once to go to the kitchen to get an extra loaf of bread and butter for the nurses. She went to the kitchen and fibbed that she needed some extra bread and butter for the patients on A3 ward. She put the food under her cape and set off to the nurses' quarters, and promptly walked into matron. She said, 'What on earth have you got under your cape?' and Mary produced the bread and butter. Mary said she was taking it to A3 ward because they had run out. Matron promptly went to the kitchen to find out what the problem was. Mary quickly scurried to her friend on the ward and told her. She emptied the bread bin and put the new loaf in. Matron then entered the ward, looked in the bread bin and found the new loaf. She 'wiped the floor' with the nurse telling her that, 'It is a disgrace, a perfect disgrace. I am not having my patients starved because of your inefficiency!' The nurse broke down in tears, but at the end of it all, Mary still went back and got the bread and butter to take to the nurses.

Joyce Escott decided to write a note in the suggestion book following an outbreak of diarrhoea among the junior nurses. They had eaten meat stew, but the senior staff ate salad with no ill effects. She suggested that the stew be served to patients with constipation. The page was, of course, removed from the suggestion book before the next meal.

Ivy McConnell remembers matron coming to the ward with a letter from a grateful patient, but the letter had a sting in its tail. It asked matron to pass on the patient's thanks to the staff of E9 ward for their kindness while he was a patient there. He wrote that they were always helpful and courteous, but added that he would like to draw matron's attention to one item, however: 'I do not think it is right for such hard-working nurses to have their meals in the patients' cloakroom. Would it not be possible for them to have time to use their canteen?' Without another word matron left the ward.

When living in, nurses always found ways of getting round the rigid rules of the nurses' home, but Gladys Tubb's friend Jean found 'breaking back in' quite a frightening experience. Late back once to the nurses' home, she found herself locked out. Not fancying the anger of the night sister who was always busy in the hospital, nor of matron the next morning, she decided to climb through a ground floor window. There was only one open. Being small in size, she thought she could get through. Part of the building that held the nurses' home was out of bounds to student nurses and they did not know the layout of that area. She climbed quietly through the window feet first and lowered herself down, touching something. Suddenly there was an enormous scream from below, and then Jean yelled as her leg was grabbed. Miss Wooton, the assistant matron, had been sitting on the toilet! Next morning Jean was summoned to see matron. Having asked Jean how she would normally enter her own home, matron said, 'Poor Miss Wooton, you nearly scared her to death!' Matron was having the greatest difficulty keeping a straight face. Many nurses had experiences of climbing over railings, crawling under windows, and creeping past the night sister to get back into the nurses' home. For Monica, a miniature whisky for the porter worked every time.

Elizabeth Bailey was more fortunate after her night out. She inadvertently fooled matron one night when coming in late. She and her friend had been to Bath to meet a couple of 'Yanks'. They spent all their money in a café and returned to the hospital very late. There was an order that if the air raid siren sounded in the daytime, the night staff would resume their duties and take the mobile patients into the shelter. The day staff would then stay with the patients, putting them and their mattresses under the beds. At night this was reversed. Elizabeth was returning from Bath as the siren sounded. 'I dashed into my room and just got my dress off when matron rushed in. "Oh," she said, "you good girl," and dashed off. She thought I had just got out of bed in response to the siren.'

Lynette King's father was not happy that his daughter was going out so much and found matron to be a suitable moral guardian. Matron Dorothy Hughes was from a Welsh coal-mining family. She was a large, buxom woman with a voice to match. She informed Mr King that his daughter's work was not affected, but if it were to become so, she would deal with it. 'From this point on, Dad affectionately called her "Dot" or "dear Dot", though not to her face may I add!' One Saturday morning, however, whilst based on the private wards, Lynette and a friend ended up in a doctor's son's room, listening to the hit parade. They were sitting on the patient's bed – a terrible crime – singing along to a song when they saw the boy's facial expression change. Turning round, they saw Matron Hughes standing there, hands on hips! This had to mean trouble: she demanded to know just what they thought they were doing, and gave them instructions to report to her office immediately. They were terrified and shaking with fear. 'Our faces must have been a picture. We were both severely reprimanded and, needless to say, I did not listen to the hit parade for a long time – and certainly did not sit on a patient's bed again!'

Mixing with the male sex was not advisable, as Josephine Chadkirk quickly learned. Each Christmas Eve, all the nurses who were not on duty had to put their cloaks on with the red side facing out, and sing carols throughout the hospital. One year, the RSO (medical officer) invited everyone to his quarters for a Christmas drink and a mince pie. It was all very innocent, but matron was horrified! She reminded him that nurses did not mix with doctors, just as nurses did not mix with porters. This rule also applied even if a member of one's own family was of a different rank. This proved most awkward for one of the nurses because her mother was a night sister. Sisters and staff nurses did not mix with junior nurses, let alone eat with them. 'Needless to say, we all managed to get around these strict rules and regulations. On the whole we were a happy, hard-working crew.'

Molly Scarth (née Hall) trained at Adelaide Hospital, Dublin. The night sister caught Molly and her friend Marjorie ten minutes after the time they were due off duty 'innocently talking to the young male patients'. Summoned before Matron next morning, they were punished by being sent home on one month's suspension. Caught between a strict matron and a traditional mother, Molly tried each morning to anticipate the dreaded letter about her 'misdemeanour'. Her explanation to her mother that she was on extra leave did not work. Her mother got the letter and immediately took Molly back to the hospital where Matron put her on a ward with a very strict Sister 'who will not put up with any of your nonsense!'

In matron's day, most nurses remembered staying on duty throughout Christmas and generally having a good time. Monica Matterson nearly had too good a time. Her matron had decreed that there would be no off-duty at all on Christmas Day. There was also to be no smoking or drinking, but the ward sister, who was normally a 'dragon of a woman', came in with a box of Player's cigarettes and some cider. She left with the warning, 'Don't let Matron catch you!' Monica neither drank nor smoked, but the nurses wanted to teach her how to inhale. She got half-way down the cigarette and had drunk a glass of cider when she suddenly felt terrible. 'Of course the ward sister found me, and instead of bawling me out she bundled me into a side room, locking the door so matron would not catch me!'

Patients were always matron's first consideration. Mr Whittaker was a porter at a royal hospital when he came out of the Royal Air Force Regiment in 1947. He found that matron's rules were in many ways more rigid than those in the armed forces. As a porter he had to man the telephones, polish the wooden floors and escort staff around the hospital, whilst being on call the whole time. The porter's job also entailed preparing patients for theatre. He was on a shift from two o'clock until ten o'clock, and, just before ten, the light flashed, signalling for a porter. He had been washing his hands prior to finishing his shift, but picked up the telephone to be told by the ward sister that there was a 'prep' that needed doing. He informed her that he was ready to leave, but that the next duty porter would be reporting for duty so he would certainly tell him. Early the next morning, he heard a knock at his front door and was surprised to find the Head Porter standing there. He said, 'Matron wants to see you immediately!' Mr Whittaker had to dress in his uniform and return to the hospital there and then. In her office, Matron looked him up and down and, with a face like thunder, said, 'As you feel your time off and your need to go home are more important than my patients, you can have two days' suspension. Dismissed!' 'That was it, I was off for two days without pay. Can you imagine that now? They should bring those ladies back!'

Although Elizabeth Bailey had a lot of respect for her matron and remembers her as a very fair woman, she did have one unfortunate occasion when she had to put herself first.

Nurses were not allowed to marry without permission, but Elizabeth and her fiancé were not planning to marry until the following June, so this should not have been a problem. However, her future husband arrived home and said he had some bad news: he was to be posted to the Far East. They were discussing the implications of this news when Elizabeth's mother said, 'You are daft. If you get married before he goes away, think of what you could save up with the Air Force allowance.' So they decided to get married by special licence. Elizabeth rang the hospital and said she wanted time off to get married. When she was put through to matron, Elizabeth asked her if she could have an extra two nights off to get married, as they normally were allowed two per month. Matron said, 'Certainly not, nurse. There is a war on, patients' needs come first.' Elizabeth's mother went with her to the hospital to talk to matron. 'Matron reluctantly agreed. She never did like her nurses to marry; it was too much of a distraction.'

Matron's insistence on putting patients first was probably just as well for one particular nurse. Billie Godfrey was acting as Sister on a medical ward in London. At the time she was managing the ward, there were a lot of refugee girls who had been encouraged to work in London hospitals. One of these girls was Polish. 'The patients were very good to us nurses, and one man was particularly helpful. He was a very timid, polite gentleman, and very keen to help us.' The Polish nurse was obviously new to the country and, having not yet had time to make any friends, was rather lonely. One day, following the patient's discharge, the nurse announced that the gentleman had contacted her and had very kindly invited her out for tea. On the day the Polish nurse was supposed to visit him, it happened that Billie was very short of staff. Appealing to matron, Billie was told that there were no extra staff available and that she would have to tell the nurse to stay on duty. Obviously the nurse was very disappointed. 'A few days later, the same man was arrested and featured on the front pages of all the newspapers. His name was John Christie! Had we saved her?' This could well have ended in disaster. On 31

March 1953, Constable T. Ledger arrested John Christie on a bridge overlooking the River Thames. Christie was the notorious resident of 10 Rillington Place, London. He befriended and murdered at least seven women, telling them he was a doctor. He would take the women to his house, give them some sort of gas, sexually assault and then murder them. Their bodies were found under the floorboards, sealed under the stairs, and buried in the garden. He went on trial for these atrocities in June 1953. He was found guilty, and executed on 15 July 1953.

Men began entering into the nursing profession in large numbers following the Second World War. This new development was met with mixed feelings from both matrons and female nurses. There was objection to them working on the wards, and of course there was the moral protection of the female nurses to consider. In psychiatric hospitals, men had already been employed for many years as nurses and orderlies, but up until the late 1960s, male and female staff, and patients, were segregated by gender.

Having left the forces in 1948 and commenced training at Wolverhampton Royal Hospital, Roy Stallard found that matron could be very helpful. He went to ask Matron Richie for advice because he was struggling economically. He explained to her how difficult it was to manage on a low income. She said he should give her a little time to think about it, and she would let him know what she could do. Two weeks later she sent for him: she had found an opportunity at Cannock Technical College. He was to teach anatomy and physiology to hairdressing students, and be paid at the technical college rate. 'I went every Monday afternoon from half past one to four, and I received a monthly cheque from then on. I was forever grateful because it eventually led to a career in nurse teaching.'

Cliff Morgan also had cause to be grateful to matron. She paid men at the orderlies' rate of wages, as they were higher than student wages. As a student working in theatre, Cliff was working late, cleaning and packing drums, when matron appeared and asked if he had had dinner. He said no, and that he had to catch the last bus home at ten. She insisted that he have something to eat, and promptly arranged for him to have supper in the dining room. Just as he finished, the hospital driver came to take him home.

Matron Richie confronted Mike Owen about his past when he was interviewed for a nurse trainee post at the Royal Hospital, Wolverhampton. 'I was just out of the army, and had been a bit of a lad when I was young. When I saw Miss Richie, a wonderful matron by the way, she said, "Any nonsense with my nurses and you will be out, Mr Owen."' Male nurses could definitely add to matron's anxiety.

Foreign nurses began to work in British hospitals from the mid-1960s onwards. They were a great addition to the skilled workforce and broadened the culture of hospital life, but by the time they were in positions to apply for matron appointments, the Salmon reorganisation had effectively ended any such opportunities. Foreign nurses have since occupied many senior nursing and management posts.

The first black matron to be appointed in Britain was Daphne Steele SRN SCM. Miss Steele was appointed Matron of St Winifred's Maternity Hospital, Ilkley in Yorkshire in 1966. On her first day she was embarrassed to be met by an array of photographers. 'It was not my qualifications that brought them, but the fact that, as a native of Guyana, I was the first coloured woman to be appointed matron of a British Hospital ... On the social side, I am constantly being asked to give talks, whether on my life or about my native land. I dreaded it at first – and still do for that matter – but if my doing this could be a means of bringing about racial tolerance then, God helping me, I'll carry on!'[1]

Matron would take a very keen interest in the welfare of her child patients, particularly at Christmas time. Janet Gilbert was in hospital in 1960 with a deep-seated abscess in her spine. This required a long period of hospital care, including the whole Christmas period. At first Janet did not like matron. When she came round, the children would be frightened to move. At Christmas, however, all of the senior staff dressed up, including matron. 'Every bed was visited, and matron wore a Minnie Mouse outfit. After that I looked at her in a completely different way. She was suddenly very human.'

Eric Cooper was a thirteen-year-old patient in the Round Block of Kendray Isolation Hospital, Barnsley. Suffering from tuberculosis, he was on a ward for children of all ages. Every morning matron made her rounds, arriving at Round Block at about eleven o'clock. The children had to be sat up in their neatly made beds, with the sheets, blankets and counterpanes tightly stretched across them. Matron would enter with her escort, namely a ward sister and one of the assistant matrons. She would take two steps inside the door and wait. This was the children's cue to sing a greeting to her, so with a nod from the ward sister, who had taught them, to the tune of 'Happy Birthday', they would sing:

> Good morning to you,
> Good morning to you.
> Good morning, dear matron,
> Good morning to you.

She would then give a smile and a curt 'Good morning, children', before carrying out her inspection. On his fourteenth birthday, Eric was classed as an adult and was now allowed to sit in a chair at the side of his bed, providing he was wearing a dressing gown and slippers. He did not have to sing to her anymore!

Note

1. 'My First Year at St Winifred's' (*Nursing Mirror*, 9 September 1966). Reproduced by kind permission of the *Nursing Times*. Little more is known about this lady, but I am grateful to Benita Fernandes for her information.

XIII

The Other Side of Matron

Matrons were human beings, they were women. They had interests apart from their careers and lived very full lives. Like everyone else, they too had relationships. Two of the matrons in the following section had fiancés who were killed in the Second World War. Had these deaths not occurred, they might well have not continued with their careers in nursing. At a time when women were beginning to establish themselves as leaders in nursing and teaching, the First World War was to deprive Great Britain of millions of men. This left a whole generation of women who had limited prospects for marriage. However, as a result, the two professions for nursing and teaching had their pick of highly intelligent, dedicated women, able and willing to devote their lives to their jobs.

Although the role of matron had originated in religious orders, most matrons had active and enjoyable social lives that did not necessarily exclude men. Matrons had never made a vow of chastity. Some matrons chose not to marry, others resigned their posts to get married, and others married only after they had retired. Nevertheless, to the young nurse, matron was often seen as an old, authoritarian spinster, unable to comprehend or remember what it was like to be young.

Mary Barnes knew that matron was well aware of the covert activities going on within her nurses' home. Mary and many of her colleagues thought that matron was a bit of a battleaxe. Because she was unmarried, they regarded her as 'a bit of an old maid'. They thought, 'How can she understand us as students? She is far too old' – but obviously she did. That was why they could get away with so little; matron had done it all herself and knew all the tricks. They did have their own system with the last nurse back closing and locking the bathroom window, but matron informed them, 'I know very well the bathroom window is used for getting in and out. It was in my day!' Nothing escaped the students' attention either. One nurse pointed out, 'Our matron was not married, but it did not stop her from having male friends and, as students, we all noticed when she did, and that was quite often.' Frances Trimmer and her nurse colleagues certainly noticed matron's behaviour, 'The matron at the hospital where I worked had a boyfriend. She always thought she was very discreet, and used to try and get him in and out without anyone noticing, but we all knew who he was and that he was married.' One nurse remembers a very different matron, who had more liberal attitudes towards men. 'She was certainly a one for the male doctors, and one of them in particular. He was called Gordon and whenever he came near her, she would sing, "A Gordon for me!" I am sure she used to frighten him to death.'

Without doubt matron was the person whom nurses felt would be there for them in moments of crisis. Matron proved to be a crucial support for Lynette King when she was struggling with exams. Matron helped her survive a period of extreme distress: her final exams were looming, and wedding arrangements for her and her fiancé had been called off. In a trembling and tearful emotional turmoil, Lynette told matron that she wouldn't and couldn't sit her state finals. Matron talked to her, and persuaded and encouraged her to put her problems in the background and not give up on what she had worked so hard for. 'Through her I did all my exams, which I passed well, and she was genuinely delighted for me. The wonderful smile she gave me on award ceremony evening said it all.'

While Chris Farmer was still at Ballochmyle, a Dutch airliner crashed near the hospital. They were woken by Matron Gillanders and told what had happened and what was expected of them. It was Gillanders who organized the surgical ward so that they could take casualties, and who freed up one ward to act as a mortuary. All that the nurses knew was that there were thirty-seven passengers on board. Of these people, there were only four survivors, and they were terribly burned. The bodies of the other passengers had to be moved to the mortuary area. 'It was terrible not being able to help these people.' Of the survivors, one or two came out of unconsciousness and the nurses thought they were going to survive, but then the patients went into shock. It was a tragic and frustrating experience; the doctors could not gain access to their veins because they kept collapsing, a result of the shock. 'Matron Gillanders was wonderful throughout, and a great support to us young nurses. Afterwards she talked about what had happened, reassured us that we had done our best and that there was nothing more that we could have done. She was our counsellor before counselling was invented.' It was the same situation when they had air raids and casualties in the night. 'Who was the first person there? Matron! Looking immaculate in her uniform. We were convinced she slept in it.'

Gladys Tubb could not consider Matron Naismith anything other than a wonderful matron and a great support. She looks back on her matron and remembers her not as a strict disciplinarian, but as 'a real captain of a very large and important liner, sailing through a sea that was extremely rough, in the early post war years'. She now wonders why matrons have earned such a reputation, because apart from certain individuals, they were not dragons but both human and humane. When times were hard, the nurses would work with matron and stay loyal to her.

Keeping up the morale of nurses in the nursing home was an important part of matron's work. Mary Verrier described her matron as a very fine woman, and a wonderful matron to work for, who was also an amateur photographer in her spare time. This matron would go across to the nurses' home, making sure that the nurses had a sandwich and a cup of tea, then she would put on her slide show. She never knew that the nurses did not want it. One day she left behind her lovely hat, and one of the girls came in parading the hat around. The nurse stood by the projector, and in matron's booming voice said, 'Come on, girls, I am going to cheer you all up. After all, you are a long way from home.' They were in hysterics, but then silence fell – watching from the half-open door was Matron. All she said was, 'I see you have my hat on, nurse. Kindly take it off!'

Matron Jones of the Eye Infirmary, Wolverhampton came from a large Irish family. Roy Stallard points out that she had lived in some grandeur in those days. The nurses' accommodation proved quite useful when the Midlands Grand National was run. Matron Jones could accommodate a number of her family in rooms vacated by nurses on leave. At this time, the General Nursing Council had decided to look at nursing accommodation around the country. While six 'guests' were ensconced, the GNC phoned to arrange a visit that Monday. Matron decided to take action against this by putting 'Night nurse sleeping, do not disturb' signs on the doors of each of the six rooms. It worked!

Ena Puncher answered an advert to be a matron's personal maid at St Mary's Hospital, Portsmouth, in 1939. She was eighteen years old. The matron in question was Miss Gay. Ena never regarded her work as a duty and thoroughly enjoyed attending to matron's needs. She found Miss Gay to be a kind, gentle and very nice person, although she could be outspoken when necessary. Having her own flat, Ena was not encouraged to mix with the other maids who were in separate rooms in the corridor above her. Her work was mainly cleaning and providing refreshments, and also looking after matron's personal needs. She did all Miss Gay's personal laundry apart from her uniform, which was always starched beautifully. She would choose what Miss Gay was to wear, whether it was for an informal social evening, an invitation to open a fête, or a ball. Miss Gay had a gas stove fitted into the bathroom so that Ena could prepare light meals. 'Every morning at eleven o'clock I would provide drinks, and even make Horlicks for the Medical Superintendent because of his weak tummy.' Although Ena had set hours, she never stuck to them, viewing her working relationship as more like a mother and daughter's relationship. 'I was there for Miss Gay in the morning, and when she retired for the evening. I used to run her bath, then tuck her up in bed and kiss her good-night!'

During the war when there were air raids, Matron Gay and Assistant Matron Miss Mansbridge would go down to the basement where Ena would have already prepared the beds. Ena would not go down herself, as she felt much safer walking the corridors until the all clear. Both Miss Gay and her replacement, Matron Sutcliffe, attended Ena's wedding. Miss Gay herself only married after she had retired, and she and Ena continued to correspond with each other for many years.

'My maid?' recalled another matron. 'My goodness, she was a tartar! She used to be very curt with other people, but never with me. I don't think she would dare, do you? I knew she used to go round with her nose in the air, thinking she was better than anyone else, but she was so good to me and looked after all of my needs. I had to have her with me because my life was so busy. She did the cleaning, got my meals, and helped with my clothes.'

The matron of a hospital was a highly respected person in the community. Miss Mary Winifred Sutcliffe (affectionately known as 'Wyn') exemplified all that was expected of this role and more. She was born in Burnley, Lancashire, on 20 October 1905. She was educated at the Skipton Grammar School for Girls, and gained management skills by taking over as manager of the cotton mills owned by her father. In June 1928, she began her training as a nurse at the St Charles Hospital, London. She undertook further training, including maternity and psychiatric nursing. Following a number of posts as sister in the north of England, she secured her first assistant matron post at St Mary's Hospital, Portsmouth. She was promoted to matron in July 1941. She was noted for being frank and outspoken, and as regards defending her nurses, it was said she had no equal. Although she did not like nurses to 'live out' ('Dreadful not knowing if they will all turn up for duty . . .'), she nevertheless appreciated having married women in the nursing work-force. 'They brought maturity and experience to the hospital.'

On the day Miss Sutcliffe was to take up the appointment of assistant matron at St Mary's Hospital, Portsmouth, she needed to employ all her powers of persuasion. The police stopped her at the top of Portsdown Hill, which overlooks Portsmouth. On 10 January 1941, the city had been ravaged by considerable bombing. She had to convince the authorities that her services were required at the hospital before they would allow her to continue her journey.

With her great zest for life, Miss Sutcliffe was able to manage an active social life alongside her duties as matron. She was an ardent cricket fan, of the Hampshire team, and also supported the Portsmouth football team. At both teams' venues, she had her own seat. For the cricket, she would even turn out in her whites, 'and bowl overarm'. She was also a proficient rally car driver, professional ballroom dancer, and an accomplished pianist. She liked nothing more than taking over the bar at the public house/hotel owned by her sister, Mrs Butterfield. Mrs Butterfield recalls, 'Because of the Second World War, my husband and I had to delay our honeymoon. Many years later we decided that we would take three weeks off as a delayed honeymoon. Wyn immediately offered and, rearranging her schedule, ran the place while we were away.'

By 1966, Miss Sutcliffe's nursing career had ended, but her civic career had just begun. In 1972, Miss Phyllis Lowe, a friend of Miss Sutcliffe's, became Lord Mayor of Portsmouth. She offered Miss Sutcliffe the position of Lady Mayoress. Miss Lowe was matron of St James Psychiatric Hospital, Portsmouth. She was a highly respected and revered lady; she put up with no nonsense, but was very fair and professional.

In 1980, Miss Sutcliffe became Lord Mayor and returned the honour by appointing Miss Lowe as her Lady Mayoress. As well as becoming Lord Mayor, she joined the Portsmouth City Council, was a Governor at Portsmouth Girls' High School, and also joined the committee of Portsmouth Polytechnic. She was also an honourary life member of the

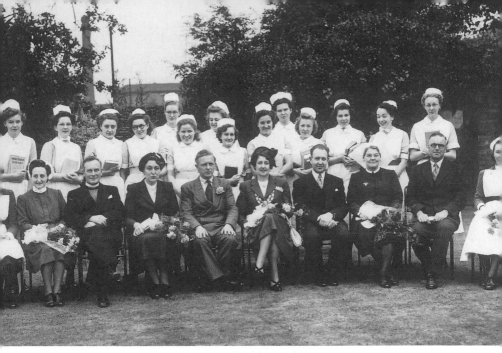

Miss Naismith, matron (*front row, third from right*), Miss Wooton, assistant matron (*front row, second from left*) and Gladys Tubb (*back row, third from left*) at Peterborough Memorial Hospital, *c.* 1950

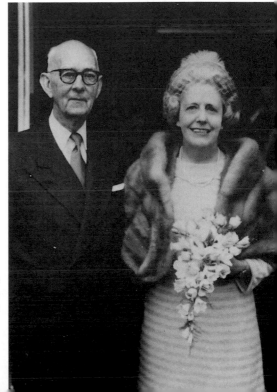

Dr Robert and Mrs Mary Rose Wrangham on their wedding day, 1978

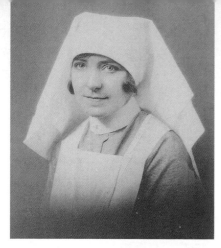

Lucy Baird on her twenty-first birthday in 1931 proudly wearing the elaborate hat of that time

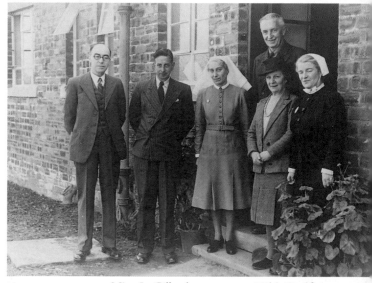

Miss J. Gillanders, matron 1946–59 (*far right*) with Miss Peterkins, sister tutor (*centre*) at the opening of the training school at Ballockmyle Hospital, Scotland

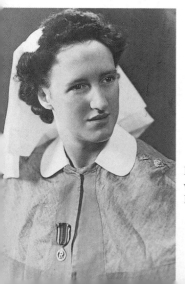

Emily Soper, in the army sister uniform she wore throughout her service in Normandy, Belgium and India 1944–7

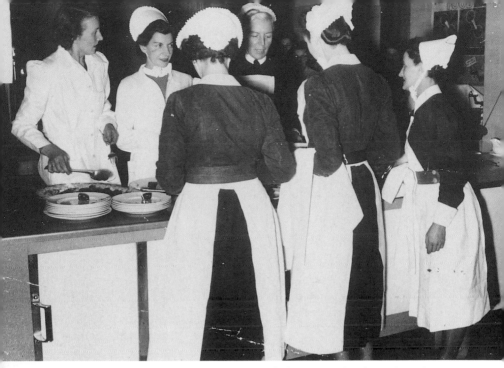

Hilda Deacon, assistant matron, in 1939, with the matron (not known) serving meals to staff to ensure that an adequate diet was had by all

Janet Baseley in bed in the children's ward, Royal Hospital, Portsmouth, Christmas 1960. Matron is dressed in the Minnie Mouse outfit

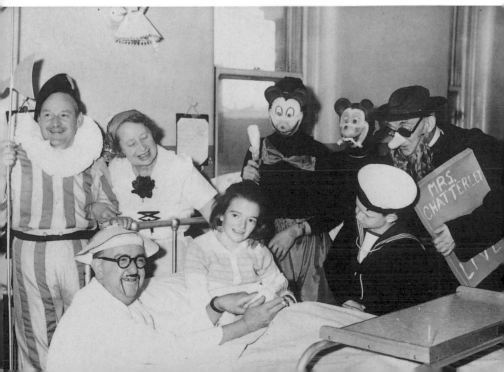

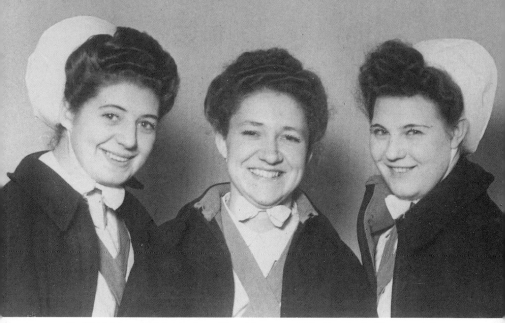

In 1944 Margaret Morris, Joan Churchhouse and Iris Cornforth, like many others, formed a lifetime bond in the nurses' home at Miller Hospital, Greenwich

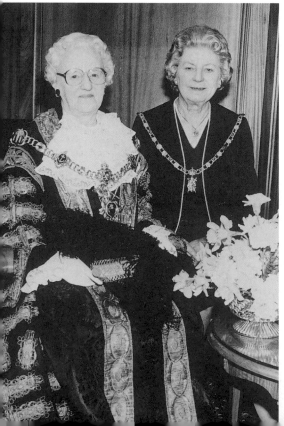

Lord Mayor Wyn Sutcliffe and Deputy Lady Mayoress Phyllis Lowe 1980–1. Both these ladies had been matrons of hospitals in Portsmouth. Miss Sutcliffe had deputized for Miss Lowe when she was Lord Mayor

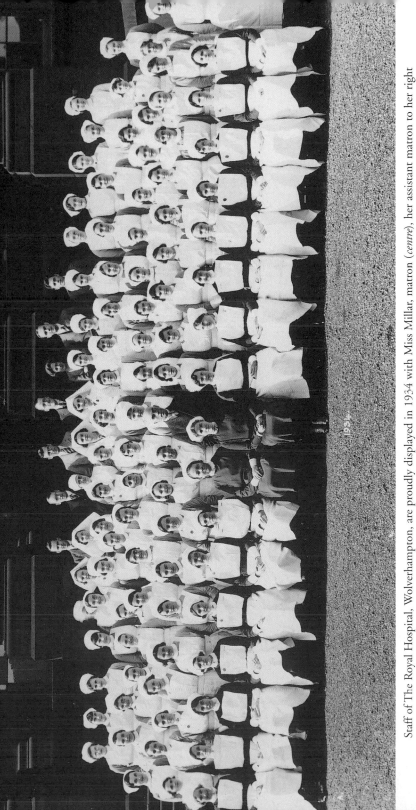

Staff of The Royal Hospital, Wolverhampton, are proudly displayed in 1934 with Miss Millar, matron (*centre*), her assistant matron to her right and Mr Norval Graham, chairman, immediately behind her

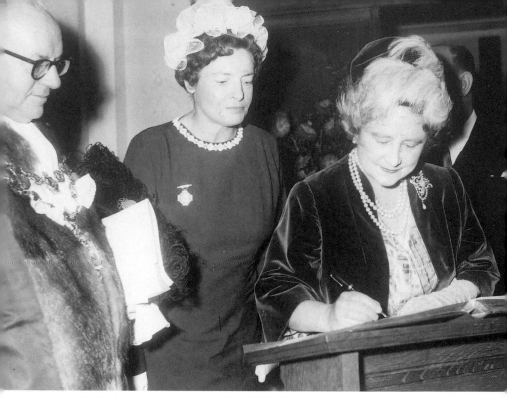

Miss Barbara Scott, matron, with HRH The Queen Mother on their second meeting at Queen Elizabeth Hospital, Birmingham, 1961

Kathleen Cooper, matron (*far right*) with Peggy Nuttall (*second from left*) editor of *Nursing Times* at a prize-giving, Bridgewater Hospital, 1969

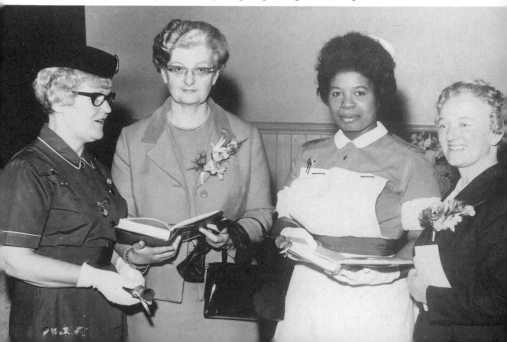

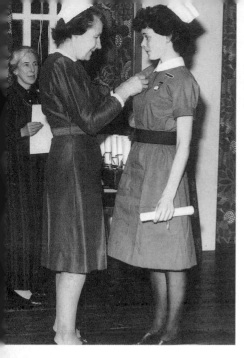

Maureen Fraser-Gamble, matron of Hammersmith Hospital, London, presents a prize to a nurse, 1980

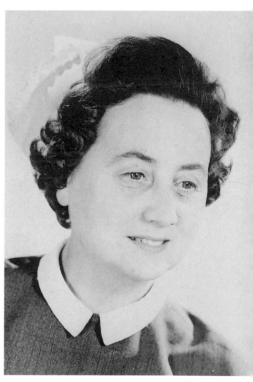

Marion Beveridge, matron of Hope Hospital, Salford, 1969

Miss Margaret Schurr, matron of Fulham Hospital, 1959. Note that, in the picture, she wears her training school University College Hospital cap, a privilege on promotion to the position of matron

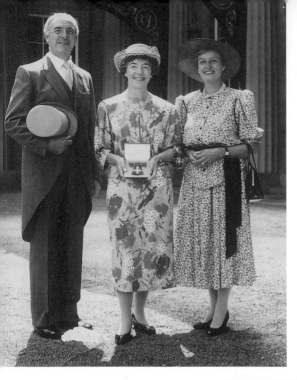

Ann Hirons, matron of Birmingham General Hospital receiving her MBE in 1987 accompanied by her brother, Dick, and sister-in-law, Ann

Miss Joyner, *c.* 1920. With so many hospitals and infirmary records having been destroyed we are often left with just a picture and a name. This lady was matron of a workhouse infirmary in Portsmouth. Nothing more is known of her

British Red Cross, and president of Portsmouth and District Soroptimists. She received the honour of 'The Freedom of the City of London' from the Queen, which allowed her the dubious honour of being able to walk her sheep through the city. This was followed by the award of the MBE in 1984, and the title of Honorary Alderman of Portsmouth in 1986. Miss Sutcliffe died in October 1992. The City of Portsmouth honoured her with a Civic Funeral on what would have been her eighty-sixth birthday.

The meeting of Emily Soper's army matron and the lady of the manor at a garden party was one occasion where matron had to show her authority and fight for her identity. The local lady of the manor (an Honourable Lady) was opening a summer fête at one of the hospitals. On the platform were the Lady, the matron of the local hospital, and the military matron in full uniform. Many of the nurses from the unit commanded by the matron were present. The Honourable Lady turned to the military matron and asked her what organization she represented. 'It's not NAAFI, is it? I am sure I know that uniform.' For a moment there was a deathly hush, then matron, resplendent as usual in her grey and scarlet, drew herself to her full height and spat, 'I am a Lieutenant-Colonel in the Queen Alexandra's Imperial Military Nursing Service, Madam!'

'We all had to muffle our laughter into handkerchiefs,' said Emily Soper.

Until 1948, nursing staff had to join in fund-raising activities to finance the voluntary hospitals. Most of the nurses found this a chore and hated it, especially the 'tin rattling'. Gladys Tubb fully understood the problems of funding. She pointed out that equipment was in extremely short supply, and very expensive. Sheets would be patched, then cut down for use as dressings, cloths, draw-sheets, theatre cloths, and eventually as cleaning rags. 'Nothing was wasted. 'Disposables' were the bits you threw away, but only when useless.'

Mary Verrier can remember when her matron was reduced to tears because of insufficient and poor equipment. Nurses seemed to be forever short of equipment and always having to go 'cap in hand'. Breakable equipment became an important issue as breakages cost money. Nurses used to host coffee mornings, help the League of Friends with whist-drives, and shake collecting tins at the ward entrance. 'We were usually ordered to go out on Flag Days – most nurses hated that. The hospital ran on voluntary funds, but we nurses often resented having to do it, especially as we were often so tired.' Assistant Matron Miss Buwick was apparently a master at fund-raising. 'You dare not leave a pair of shoes around or they would end up in a jumble sale. They did not care what they did because it was for the patients.' A nurse had to be careful about what she left in her room since it could disappear into the jumble – or worse! Joyce left her father's hat on her bed, ready to put in the jumble, but it nearly cost her her job! The assistant matron was doing a round of the nurses' home and found the hat on her bed. This was immediately reported to matron who sent for the nurse and demanded an explanation. 'What is a man's hat doing in your room, nurse?' Joyce's explanation was accepted, but only after a great deal of convincing.

Many matrons had pets, often dogs. The pets could have pride of place anywhere in the hospital. In matron's office they would often have a corner under her desk. It was extremely important to be accepted by the pet. Lucy Baird was so fond of Matron Radford's dog, Billy, that she would take him on her rounds when she was district nursing. For Derek McCarthy, a future divisional nursing officer, helping matron's pet proved to be a good beginning to his nursing career. He was working on the neurology ward, his first placement. During his first week, at one point he was cleaning out some glass syringes by the window and gazing out, 'as one does', at a torrential rainstorm. In the road he saw a big, long-haired dog. It was there at nine in the morning, looking very bedraggled, barely moving, just standing there. On and off he watched it, and it still just stood there. It was cold weather in Newcastle. When he went off duty, he checked the collar of the dog and found its name and address. It did not have a lead, so as he had a big duffel coat with toggles and a hood, he decided the only thing he could do was to wrap the poor dog up in it and carry it. As he squeezed the dog to his chest, it dripped water all down him, but still Derek staggered off down the street, carrying this dog with him. Having walked for about a quarter of a mile, he found a large Victorian house. He walked up the drive and rang the bell. The door was opened and he could not believe his eyes when he saw that the occupant was his matron. By this time Derek was soaking wet, and the poor dog was bedraggled. The first thing that struck him was that matron was still wearing her green uniform, but the top was open. It was a uniform that buttoned up to the shoulder. She had obviously been getting changed, as the top was undone right down the front, exposing her petticoat. He thought it most unusual to see matron looking like that, and she made no attempt to cover herself up. She saw the dog and her eyes lit up. She said, 'Oh, that is my dog! I have been looking everywhere for him. I did not know where he was and he is nearly blind.' She knew Derek worked at the hospital, but she never mentioned it again.

At the end of his training, Derek had to report to matron. He was standing in the usual line outside her office, and when it came to his turn he told her that he had sat his exams and was due to go back to the mental illness hospital. 'She asked, "Would you like a charge nurse's post in the department of psychological medicine?" I wondered if this went back to the episode with the dog. I told her that I would love it, so she suggested that I write to her when I passed, and assured me that I would have a post.'

In 1927 Matron Booth at the Isolation Hospital, Preston, had a pet, a black spaniel called Dash. Dash was an important part of the hospital. If he was happy, all was well! Every year for his birthday a bag would be hung at the bottom of the staircase for subscriptions. When Dash died a patient on the fever ward penned the following poem:

IN MEMORY OF DASH

Here lies the body of dear old Dash,
Who departed this life without a splash.
He rambled and growled around the IHP grounds,
But never appeared in the Lost and Found.

His tombstone was erected with subs from the nurses,
Who gave the money with numerous curses.
They parted with it, one desire to atone
For wishing that Dash hadn't gone alone.

Missed will he be by Lady Booth
For now she has nothing to soothe.
Oh! Dash, why did you go when looking so well?
Are you in heaven . . .?

Although you are buried within sight of the Home,
Your mistress will often think of a bone.
All bones are now reserved for the staff.
So, Dash, while you sleep so cold in the grave,
The nurses remember your funny ways
And to keep you so fresh in our memory
We think of Matron RIP.

When matron donned her uniform it was as if she were slipping into a persona, a role, and a heritage. In this uniform she would present a powerful, confident and competent image that seeped into her bones, sometimes masking the sensitive woman beneath. However, a matron's family and friends would remember the softer side of her.

Trained at Paddington Hospital in 1927, Hilda Deacon became assistant matron at the Royal Sussex Hospital, Brighton. Later she was to become matron of the Darvell Hall Sanatorium, Robertsbridge, and then of the Royal Hospital for Consumptives, Ventnor, Isle of Wight. Her references (all written between 1935 and 1944 by medical superintendents) speak of Hilda as an intelligent, careful and active person with impeccable dress standards 'and a real passion for her work'. She was also painstaking in the teaching of her staff, and her success as matron is eloquent testimony to her work. Despite her undoubted success as a matron she sometimes talked to her family about loneliness of her job. The Deacon family found 'Aunt Hilda' to be a very different woman when she retired from her matron post. Betty

Deacon, her sister-in-law, found that

> She even talked different, less starchy! Where Hilda had been
> a no-nonsense matron who would not spare the rod, she was
> so gentle and kind within the family. While matron she could
> be quite curt at times, and even seemed a little aloof to us, but
> when she retired we saw such a different, warm side to her.
> Her brother Jack, my husband, was the only one she would
> ever cry in front of. He was very proud of her.

She was always Aunt Hilda to Ray, her nephew. A lady who
could command the room whenever she was present, Hilda
would sit at the bottom of the stairs with Karen, Ray's step-
daughter, and help her with her school-work. Ray recalls:

> I remember being taken as a child by my aunt round the Royal
> Sussex Hospital on Christmas Day. We had a close relation-
> ship and so she took me with her as she visited every ward. I
> was very proud! I always kept in touch with her by regular
> visits. When I was preparing to marry Janet, she insisted on
> accompanying her to choose the wedding dress. Janet really
> appreciated this, but Aunt Hilda had such taste in fashion and
> we were so tight for money at the time, she had to turn the
> offer down.

Libby, a neighbour and friend, had great respect for her.
'Hilda was always immaculate, whether in her uniform or out
shopping, and she loved her shopping. She always looked like
a model. With her pet dog, of whom she was very fond, she
would be out walking most days.'

On retirement from the health service, Miss Deacon started
a second career in beauty and fashion at Hannington's department store in Brighton. She took a course with Lancôme
perfumes and, not surprisingly, soon took over the beauty
department of the store, and later the whole fashion department.

Like some other matrons, Miss Deacon was involved in a
secret relationship. Hers lasted for over twenty years.

Although the relationship was known to the family, there was no likelihood of marriage as the gentleman concerned was already married. In this way Miss Deacon lived a sort of double life; on the one hand, she was a proud and powerful matron, and on the other she remained a mistress in a situation that could never be resolved. Not sure if she wanted more than this from her life, she nevertheless appeared happy and satisfied with the course her life had taken. Marriage and love often came late in life to women who had devoted their lives to nursing. Nevertheless, success and happiness were important goals in life to be attained and treasured.

All that Mary Rose Wrangham (née Ellis) had ever wanted to do was to be a nurse. Her mother respected this so they went to see Miss Clieve, matron at the Royal Liverpool Children's Hospital. Too young to start formal training, Mary Rose was told that she could start working at a hospital for convalescing children in the Wirral. There, she found Matron Miss Tweed a terrifying figure, who always seemed to be on duty and was meticulous about everything. No men at all were allowed in the nurses' home and Miss Tweed would vet any boyfriends. She also made them meet the nurses at the home, and then bring them back safely. 'Mind you, Matron Tweed would comb my hair before I went on duty at eight every morning. I had very long hair and, rather than make me have it cut, she would comb it so it would go under my hat.'

At the age of eighteen, Mary Rose returned to the Royal Children's Hospital, Myrtle Street, to complete her certificate in the nursing of sick children. At this time her father became ill, and so Mary Rose looked after him at home until he died. She then went to the Queen Elizabeth Hospital, Birmingham, to complete her SRN training in 1948. After experience as a staff nurse, she went on to do her Part One midwifery at the London Hospital, and Part Two at Oxford. This was followed by an application to join the Princess Mary's Royal Air Force Nursing Service. She wanted to travel and found the idea of flying terribly exciting, and ten long weeks later, she received a letter saying, 'Her Majesty has the pleasure of offering you a Commission'. It was to be another two years before she did start travelling, and only because she knew the Commanding Officer (CO) that she eventually got an overseas posting. 'It was quite funny really. The matron kept tearing up my letters requesting for overseas posting. After the third time the CO, who had helped me write them, advised me to get an appointment with the visiting Matron-in-Chief.' She did, and after talking to Dame Mary Williamson she got her posting. 'Matron got her own back. She made me buy her 'overseas hat' for ten shillings. It was originally bought at Boyd Cooper in London. The posting was to Egypt at the time of the Suez crisis.'

A posting to Cyprus followed, this time during a period of terrorist warfare. Mary Rose worked mainly with the army nurses. Her matron was Colonel Fitzpatrick, 'a wonderful woman'. They had many opportunities to fly in Cyprus; on one of the flights she had to escort a three-day-old baby to Great Ormond Street Hospital. She was suffering from congenital duodenal atresia, a fatal condition in those days. The baby was as tiny as a bag of sugar, and during the ten-hour flight to England she needed intravenous saline and subcutaneous feeding. Luckily the tiny infant survived her ordeal.

As a flight officer, under Group Captain Jackson, Miss Ellis helped pioneer the first kidney and dialysis unit at RAF Halton in 1959. She left the air force and started working on cruise liners as ship's nursing sister. Her first ship was the *Britannic* on the American crossing, a twenty-one day cruise. This was followed by a three-month cruise on the *Reina Del Mar*, a ship of the Pacific Steam Navigation Company. It was a very busy time on the ship because most of the passengers were either elderly or recovering from illness. There were lots of medicines to sort out and many of the guests were in bad shape.

On the SS *Reina Del Mar*, she met her future husband, Robert George Heskoth Wrangham. She was the sister and he was the doctor. After three months together, arriving in Jamaica, he said, 'I suppose you know I have fallen in love with you.' Mary Rose replied, 'Yes, and you can join the queue. I do not like the idea of a relationship with a married man. If you are ever free, you can contact me then!' And that is what he did – twenty years later. In the intervening time he travelled the world many times, and sent her a card from every place he visited. On one side it would have her name and address, and on the other three dots, depicting that he still loved her and that the flame was still burning. 'That had to keep me going, but I did not stand still waiting. I got on with my life.'

Mary Rose continued to cruise for three years and then joined QARNNS from 1962 until 1966. They had wanted experienced midwives to open a unit in Malta, and she thought it would be nice to get away from the English weather. After four years she left the navy to take an appointment as Assistant Matron at the Children's Hospital, Birmingham. She was there for over thirteen years. 'I would have taken a matron post, but opportunities were limited. It was dead men's shoes, then with the advent of Salmon, the structure changed, and that put an end to that ambition. I became a Nursing Officer.'

After the death of his wife, Robert phoned Mary Rose and asked her to meet him for dinner at St Bartholomew's Hospital. There, he proposed to her. It was 1978, she was fifty-two and he was eighty-two. He gave her two rings; one was the real one, and the other was a replica. 'That is your washing-up ring!' he told her.

'So I had my uniform on with a pocket on either side, and nurse would come and ask, "Can I see your washing-up ring?" and I would say, "Of course, look in here." No one at the hospital could have guessed, as no one knew. As far as the staff were concerned, I was the assistant matron and matrons did not marry. It was totally out of the blue, you see, so I gave one month's notice and that was that.' It was strange when they got married; they spent a lot of time getting to know each other and sharing what each had been doing during those intervening years. 'There was such a lot to catch up on! I had seven of the most wonderful years of my life.'

In about 1920, as a young man, Dr Wrangham started the

South American missionaries. He was in South America for ten years. He started a school, a chapel and a small farm. On return to England in 1930, he commenced (and paid for) his own medical training at St Mary's Hospital in Paddington. A remarkable man, he was loved by everyone and was a Christian in every sense. He performed the medical examinations free for the missionary staff. When he arrived in Chile on the SS *Reina Del Mar*, there were so many people to meet him and thank him. Robert's name was chosen to be the next High Sheriff for the County of Middlesex. This is a formal event, known as 'pricking'. Three names are put forward, and the Queen 'pricks' the one chosen.

Mary Rose had started learning how to work with porcelain in 1971, as a hobby. Now that she was married, her husband Robert encouraged her into a second career – porcelain restoration. Robert was aware of his age and that Mary Rose had given up her nursing career, so he was concerned that she might 'go potty' in their flat after his death. For these reasons, he encouraged her to set up a studio. It proved to be very successful, with a correspondence course and educational videos. Marriage and porcelain had certainly changed her life.

At seventy-five years of age, Mary Rose Wrangham is still working full-time at her studio. She is also doing a two-year course in ceramic conservation in order to obtain a Diploma, now required by new European regulations.

Norma Moore is secretary of a nurse retirement association. She told me about the 'other side of matron'. Known affectionately to her staff as Emma, Matron Elizabeth Ashton was always immaculately presented on duty, and elegant off duty. She lived in a flat attached to the hospital and would entertain senior members of staff at Christmas. She was also regularly invited to civic functions and parties. She was a well-respected member of society and knew all her nursing staff personally. Each nurse had to report to her both before and after they took leave. The same rule applied when they returned from sick leave. In this way she kept contact with her nurses, and her main interest was their welfare. She would personally take control of hospital functions, and was the first to join in the fun. The Annual Ball was a big occasion, with everyone in full evening dress. Tickets were collected from her office, and the name of one's guest had to be submitted prior to this. 'Emma' would write it on the ticket herself.

When organizational changes affected the NHS, and matron posts were lost, Miss Ashton insisted on wearing her uniform and retaining her title. 'Respecting her staff, she expected respect in return – and she got it. They all knew she would support them. You would certainly sum her up as "Captain of her own ship", with old-fashioned discipline and old-fashioned values, but also with a modern attitude to life. She was a good listener, and, like an "elephant", did not forget anything.'

Sheila Clark, Frances Trimmer and Betty Groves discussed their memories of training and found they had more to laugh about than cry over. They all agreed that they had loved their student days. Living in the nurses' home, they worked hard and, at times, felt as if they were used as 'slave labour', but, 'Our hospitals would not have been so well run or as much fun if we had not had the "old-fashioned" matron.' Despite the close supervision, nurses still managed to flirt with the doctors, have their New Year and Christmas drinks, and play tricks on whomever they could, but they knew matron was always there, keeping the hospital together and creating a safe framework in which they did their work. 'If matron ever knew what went on behind her back, we, and more than half her staff, would have been fired there and then.' Probably not, according to the matrons in the following chapter – they had seen it and done it all themselves before!

This brief look at the 'other side' of matron presents a picture of women who were able both to enjoy their work, and also to combine it with other activities. They were not the stuffy spinsters of stereotype, but professionals who were willing to commit themselves to their work without reservations. With a shortage of men suitable for marriage, and a society that promoted 'family values' and discouraged success for women in the world of careers, matrons were isolated. Women were compelled to choose between marriage or a career, and a few managed to achieve both. A matron was not in the same situation as other women and, as such, became an ideal target for largely unjustified criticism.

XIV

Nurse Leadership: A Singular Occupation

In the previous chapters, we captured the essence of matron's life, and the qualities that set her apart. Matron was the pre-eminent person in hospital life. She was the one with the presence, who could impose order on doctors, nurses, patients and relatives, such was the awe and esteem she was held in. It was matron who could deal directly with problems and solve them, and it was matron around whom the staff rallied in times of crisis. Despite having enormous resilience and adaptability, matrons could not however resist the tide of managerial and administrative changes that swamped the organization. Matrons were ultimately swept out of the corridors and wards.

In this chapter we shall see if these same qualities remain intact in a matron's later years. Six retired matrons tell their stories; none of these women consider themselves to be nursing legends; in fact they all say that they knew of matrons who were far more qualified for the title than them. Nevertheless, along with the nursing predecessors, these women have become a part of history, and they now represent a dwindling group of very fine nursing professionals, the last of their kind. Dedicated to their work, they personified all that was good about the distinctive role of matron as a nurse leader.

Through the generosity of these women, the information included in this chapter captures the reality of becoming a matron, and living as one. Starting on the bottom rung of the nursing ladder, they were exposed to the same hardships and joys as any other nurse. They worked long hours, endured the tedium of bedpan and temperature rounds, cleaned the sluice rooms, tended to pressure areas, held the hands of dying patients, and shared all the other experiences of traditional bedside nursing. They were moulded by a unique blend of their own qualities as people, and grass-roots training.

Cliff Morgan was in the best position, as a nurse educator, to observe matron in action. Mr Morgan retired as Director of Nursing and Midwifery Education in Cardiff. He saw both sides of matron – the consummate professional and the actress. His descriptions are full of admiration; he recalls matron having an iron will when fighting for resources and enforcing discipline, but also compassion and courtesy towards others. The switch between the two was often instant. To him, matron was the great ambassador of nursing, her poise, dignity and authority unsurpassed.

Before the Second World War, opportunities for women in the workplace continued to be restricted. Secretarial, teaching, or nursing positions were the most usual options. Nurses, and particularly nurse leaders, were still very much selected from 'good' families. However more openings into the profession began to emerge with the Second World War, as it lent a sense of urgency to nurse recruitment.

Matron Miss Barbara Scott commenced boarding-school at the age of ten at Queenswood School, Hatfield. She found she struggled more than her classmates at academic work, but fared much better at the more practical aspects of schooling. Her dyslexia was discovered late, and widespread ignorance of the condition meant that academic work was a frustrating experience for her, however, it was already clear that she would build on her organizational skills. With firm roots in her family and the church, Barbara learned another way of life, how to put herself in another person's position, to accept graciously, and to give without effort. Her father, a radical thinker for his time, encouraged self-sufficiency in all his children, irrespective of gender, so she took the opportunity to widen her skills. She learned farming, including poultry husbandry, and took a course in domestic science to prepare for whatever career she would choose. Still too young to start formal training as a nurse, she was keen to develop her skills with people, and an offer made to her to train as a corsetière seemed an ideal opportunity. This opportunity arose because the corsetière was fitting her mother at home. She took instruction, was set up with a bag, and off she went. It was in this way at a very tender age, that she learned a valuable trade, a business way of life, and how to communicate. Encouraged by her sister, a hospital physiotherapist, Miss Scott switched to a career in nursing. She commenced her training at Middlesex General Hospital in 1938.

Matron Miss Maureen Fraser-Gamble also experienced a somewhat unconventional education, dipping into countries and cultures as her army family moved between India, Egypt and England. Whilst in England, she was mostly educated in a convent. Now settled for a life in London, despite the vast and varied experience that travelling had given her, Miss Fraser-Gamble was uncertain about her future when she left school. The family intended for her to become a secretary, but this only galvanized her thinking. 'A secretary? Certainly not, I want to be a nurse!' So nursing it was. She commenced training at St Mary's Hospital, Paddington in 1938.

Like Miss Fraser-Gamble, Matron Miss Marian Beveridge also made her own decision to go into nursing. Born in Burnbank, Lanarkshire, in 1921, Miss Beveridge had been determined from a very young age to pursue her ambition to nurse. She sent for brochures from many hospitals in Scotland and England, and eventually chose Stobhill General Hospital, Glasgow. In those days, matrons felt it was important to see what the nurse looked like before she was accepted for interview, so Miss Beveridge had to enclose a photograph with the application. 'As students, we held matron in great esteem and had much respect for her. Though very strict and expecting high standards, she treated everyone with fairness and courtesy. Lessons I learned and remembered my whole career.'

Both Miss Fraser-Gable and Miss Beveridge, along with

Miss Scott, entered the nursing profession with clear motivation, with the intention of commencing an enduring career. Each of these women was drawn from the 'good' families on which nursing traditionally relied, so too was Matron Miss Margaret Schurr. She came from a medical family, and although there was no expectation that she would follow in family footsteps, it was the recruitment drive for the war effort which pressed her to make a decision. She was one of a group of young women for whom career decisions were accelerated by the advent of war. Having to register for war work, she became a wartime student nurse at University College Hospital in London, her home city.

From very different beginnings, but also via the war effort, Matrons Miss Kathleen Cooper and Miss Yvonne Mullin managed to follow their hearts into nursing. Miss Cooper had an unsettled childhood and left school at fourteen, at a time when the country was tentatively speculating the end of the depression. Her father, a labourer, worked at the local tannery, and she and her siblings followed suit. Her route out of the factory came when she had to register for National Service in 1939; she commenced work in the Royal Ordnance Factory in Chorley. It was here where she progressed towards her future career of nursing, when she moved from shell-filling to first aid. The nurse sister encouraged her to undertake nurse training.

Following the death of her father when she was only twelve years old, Miss Mullin was raised by her mother. It was hard for one-parent families in those days, but despite the early difficulties, her mother still managed to have her educated at a high school in Manchester. She left at seventeen with a school certificate, and she knew she could not stay much longer in fairness to her mother. So, in 1942, she elected to make her contribution to the war effort in the form of nursing.

All of these aspirant nurses started their training within eight years of one another, between 1935 and 1943. In many ways their experiences are remarkably similar. They each talk of an instant sense of responsibility during their training period; for example, Miss Cooper arrived in the Bury Infirmary, Lancashire, at three-thirty in the afternoon. She was on duty on the wards by four, and finished at nine. 'I had not a clue what I was doing!' Miss Cooper also referred to the enormous pressure placed upon them as students. Only three months into her training, she had to juggle the demands of the night shift with daytime lectures, a truly exhausting situation. 'I was only three months into my training when I was put on night duty. In the daytime I still had to go for lectures. One day I had the greatest difficulty keeping awake when the chest physician came to lecture. All I heard from him was 'Chest diseases', and that was that; I never heard another word!'

The tutors and matrons these nurses met during training left an indelible impression on them. The great author Evelyn C. Pearce, who taught Miss Scott, is remembered for her powerful character and sense of fairness. Miss Fraser-Gamble had the good fortune to be trained at St Mary's Hospital under the 'wonderful and remarkable matron' Mary Milne, the daughter of the first doctor appointed to Dr Barnardo's. Mary Milne is described as a lady, a great nurse and matron, and an inspiration to her staff. Clearly, when our matrons were students they had complete and utter respect for their matrons, understanding and respecting the need for strict rules. They knew that without these rules the patients' heath, both physical and emotional, would suffer, and the esteemed profession of nursing, of which they were so proud, would be compromised.

The ranking system familiar to these matrons, often known as the nurse hierarchy, was felt to engender inter-nurse respect. It helped to ensure that everyone knew their place and what was expected of them at each point in their career development. Teaching fitted neatly into this system, with first-year students performing the more menial tasks and learning the essentials of basic nursing, such as bedside care and the importance of ward cleanliness. The second year of their training would consolidate their knowledge and gradually increase their levels of confidence. All the trainee nurses started in a lowly position, then steadily built up their knowledge and skills, and eventually became staff nurses. By the time an appointment to Sister, or even Matron rank, was made, the appointee had gone through everything that even the most junior nurse had to. They had been through the same system, and could be proud of their achievements.

Miss Fraser-Gamble views her training as an irreplaceable nursing experience. She and her peers radiate a deep love of nursing, a belief in the validity of all they were taught and how they were taught. 'I loved every day of my training and nursing life. It is not looking back through rose-coloured spectacles, it is the truth. I just loved it. Nursing was strict, but as I had had, like most people of that time, a strict upbringing, I adjusted quite easily.' With a pride unparalleled in other vocations, our matrons were taught to be self-reliant, responsive, responsible, and completely devoted to the needs of their patients.

As she was too young to commence nurse training, Miss Mullin started her nursing career as one of six domestic pupils at the Bradford Royal Infirmary where the Lady Superintendent responsible for the infirmary had trained at the Nightingale School. As domestic pupils, they worked for a few months in the nurses' home, then the catering stores and diet kitchen, supervised all the time by an assistant matron or administrative sister. This eclectic approach provided them with not only a good grounding in hospital administration before they started their nurse training, but also gave them an advantage for the rest of their careers.

With their general training completed, most of our newly qualified nurses continued with additional training. Choosing the right course was an essential part of creating a structure of experience on which to build one's career. Miss Scott gained her state registration and, in her fourth year, became a junior staff nurse. It was usual for nurses at teaching hospitals to continue for a fourth year in order to be awarded the 'much coveted' hospital certificate. Having the certificate enabled Miss Scott to further her training with courses on tropical diseases, midwifery, health visiting, and industrial nursing.

Miss Fraser-Gamble, Miss Schurr, Miss Cooper and Miss Beveridge also continued their studies, with midwifery being the main certificate. With this certificate, they gained invaluable experience on the wards, in the delivery rooms, and in the community. Following her midwifery training, Miss Cooper was awarded a scholarship at Manchester to undertake health visitor training, but it was not 'free training' by any means – in return she was required to stay for two years. It was thought at the time that a nurse would not be able to advance without the midwifery certificate, but Miss Mullin was unfortunate to fall ill during her training and was not able to continue. Nevertheless she managed to build a successful career for herself. At this point, our six nurses embark on their own distinct paths, their futures being marked by differing opportunities and adventures.

One such adventure was the advent of war. The war was beginning just as Miss Scott finished her training in 1939. As the bombs began to fall, she decided to take a post as Sister-in-Charge of a large armament factory. 'I thought it would provide a different experience, where I could see life from the inside – I did.' Here she saw real life in all its gory details. There were endless serious accidents: girls without head-scarves for protection scalped by fast-moving machinery; a professional organist who worked on a press machine and pushed in a plate, letting the machine drop before he had removed his fingers. 'There were so many tragedies like this. It was a sickening waste.'

After two years Miss Scott returned to hospital life where she worked as a junior night sister, then as a night superintendent, before she took a ward sister post. Here, she was quickly given the opportunity to show her organizational potential when a flu epidemic struck the local community, shortly to be followed by a serious fire in the hospital!

The war proceeded, and preparations for evacuation commenced. Miss Scott was told by matron to have her trunk packed and ready in twenty-four hours. She was to leave under a heavy veil of secrecy. When the time came, Miss Scott and two other sisters joined a small group of nurses, still not knowing where they were to end up! It turned out to be Halsar Hospital, Gosport, and awaiting them was the carnage of Normandy. When the nurses lifted the injured from the stretchers to the beds, sand from the beaches was everywhere. So many men arrived, with such dreadful injuries. They were wheeled across the grass on trolleys and into the kitchen, where doctors operated using only the light from hurricane lamps.

Miss Beveridge went one step further than Miss Scott and actually joined the services. In the Queen Alexandra's Imperial Military Nursing Service, she held the rank of Lieutenant. She recalls the quality of the uniforms, which were grey and red, tailor-made by Austin Reed, and looking very smart. The nurses were required to pay for their uniforms, and they thought at the time that it was a hefty price to pay. Along with twelve other nurses, they were transferred to Netley Hospital, Southampton. Miss Beveridge found basic training and instruction in military protocol highly entertaining. When the nurses had been supplied with essential equipment, had their photographs taken for identity purposes and had portraits sent to relatives, they were then to complete their wills. This generated considerable amusement amongst the nurses, since all they had to leave behind was a set of bills for the expensive uniforms! In keeping with other military operations at the time, fifty of the nurses, including Miss Beveridge, set off by train with absolutely no idea of their destination. Boarding the liner *Reno Del Pacifico*, their voyage proceeded without incidents until they reached the Mediterranean Sea, where they were heavily bombarded. Although heartily shaken, they reached Port Said with tangible relief.

Their destination turned out to be India, and on reaching Bombay they were given their postings. Miss Beveridge and two other nurses were sent to the 39th Indian General Hospital at Midnapur in north-east Bengal. The hospital accommodated both British and Indian patients, but it was to be an uncomfortable time for the nurses. The nurses' accommodation consisted of bamboo huts. Although there were one or two stone buildings, much of the hospital was also fabricated from bamboo. The nurses quickly had to accustom themselves to different food and learn some basic Urdu. Unfortunately, shortages of food supplies in the area were adding to the prevalent anti-British feeling, and several British officials had already been assassinated. This left the nurses feeling nervous and insecure, but they did everything they could to adapt to their new environment.

The hospital received convoys of patients from Burma, and RAF patients from the surrounding camps. The climate proved to be a most terrible and relentless adversary. Heat exhaustion caused many RAF mechanics to collapse, and each day thirty or forty patients would arrive requiring emergency treatment to replace great loss of fluids and to reduce their very high temperatures. The nurses were able to boast with pride that not a single patient was lost, 'a great effort!' An American general who went to visit the hospital was so impressed by how the British nurses coped in such conditions, that he sent over some American nurses to witness for themselves. They had been giving him such a hard time that he wanted them to realize how fortunate they were – it apparently worked!

Mindful that the Japanese were threatening invasion, it was thought advisable to move many of the casualty stations and hospitals to the south of India in Bangalore. There, and in relative safety, a tented field hospital was set up, but there were no resources and no facilities, not even electricity! Miss Beveridge had arrived at the most seriously deprived hospital environment she was ever to experience. Later, Miss Beveridge was posted to a large military hospital at Secunderabad that seemed almost luxurious by comparison. The standards were exceptionally high, everything was meticulously scrutinized, not only the cleanliness of the ward, but also the nursing and medical care of patients.

For Miss Schurr, the war came crashing into England. She was a wartime student nurse at University College Hospital in 1943. Following three months in a preliminary training school, the students were placed in 'sets', and they became one of the first groups to train in a 'block system'. Because of the war there were no domestic staff, except a few daily women and conscientious objectors, so from the start there was an emphasis placed on maintaining hygiene standards, and domestic duties were designated each morning. Because of the bombing in London, the 'set' was transferred to a sector hospital, a large converted house. Many trained nurses had been drafted to the forces, so like other people in wartime, they had to be prepared to undertake some tasks that were beyond their ordinary experience. Returning to London in that June of 1944, just three days after the D-Day landing, the spirits of the nurses were inevitably high – the war seemed to be coming to an end. However, only days after their return, a flying bomb shattered Tottenham Court Road. The resultant carnage was a truly harrowing ordeal for such young and inexperienced nurses. Caring for casualties who were badly injured left an indelible mark on Miss Schurr and her nurse colleagues.

Again, the nurses were sent away to a sector hospital for safety, this time to a stately home. The grounds were littered with Nissen huts, each one catering for forty patients. The ward sisters came from different hospitals, and some were from the Queen Alexandra's Imperial Military Nursing Service. Among the wounded and sick soldiers were both British and German prisoners of war. With only eighteen months of training behind them, the nurses were left in charge of wards at night, with the help of only one auxiliary. In February 1945, they had to weather the bombing once again when they returned to their London hospital for their final state examinations.

Everyone suffered during the war, including the nurses, whether they were directly involved with tending the sick and injured, or had loved ones involved in the fighting. Our matrons were no exception; the experience of war changed them, as it did everyone else. For Miss Schurr and her colleagues, the demands of war helped them become self-reliant, to be aware that their contribution mattered, and that they had to respond, no matter what. If faced with a challenge, they prepared themselves and did not expect everything to be handed out to them. This experience encouraged a questioning and thoughtful approach to their work, and to the needs of patients.

At the end of the war, Miss Scott thought about the next stage of her career. To apply for a top post she first needed wider experience. After two years as sister of outpatients, then three years as ward sister, and four years as night superintendent, she was appointed Office Sister dealing with new candidate papers, nursing, midwifery, occupational health, physiotherapy, and general help.

Miss Mullin felt compelled to take a career path that even she found surprising. After completing her state registration, she remained a staff nurse for some time until she saw an advertisement. It was for a staff nurse position at Christie Hospital, Manchester. This hospital specialized in cancer treatments. Cancer care and care of the terminally ill were not considered 'fashionable' areas of nursing; indeed it was difficult for the hospital to attract staff. However, the Christie hospitals in London and Manchester, and the hospice movement, radically changed attitudes to this highly rewarding area of nursing. Miss Mullin applied for the position, intending to work there only for a few weeks, but she found it so inspiring that she stayed. With rapid promotion to ward sister, her time at the hospital was amongst the most satisfying of her career; however, as much as she enjoyed it, she felt she had the potential to go further, so she applied for a one-year secondment to the Royal College of Nursing for a Diploma in Nursing Administration. On return to Christie Hospital, her original post had been filled, so while she waited for a suitable position to arise, she accepted a short-term appointment of home sister where she was responsible for the supervision of the hospital accommodation. She would later return to Christie as the matron.

At the age of twenty-five, Miss Schurr was appointed ward sister of a female surgical ward where she spent five happy years. She was fortunate in this position, as she was given considerable freedom to organize the nursing care as she thought best. Very dependent on student nurses, she began to question the practice of task assignment, and would often delegate the total care of an ill patient to one or two nurses. She found that they enjoyed this and felt more involved and fulfilled. In 1956, Miss Schurr achieved the position of assistant matron at a small hospital in Woolwich. Here, she was responsible to one of the first Group Matrons. Miss Schurr had a mixture of respect and fear for this formidable lady. The group matron thought that her job in life was to prepare promising candidates for matron posts, and she taught them the hard way. Miss Schurr quickly learned how to scan reports and absorb essential details to provide matron with speedy information. She also learned not to telephone group headquarters without first thinking through the problem thoroughly. Miss Schurr clearly remembers phrases that matron would quote. One, in particular, influenced her philosophy. It referred to the corruption of power, and was attributed originally to Mary Parker Follett, 'Power *with* is more important than power *over*.'

Following her wartime experiences, Miss Scott was told by her matron that it was time for her to apply for matron posts. The response to her applications was encouraging, and after a few weeks she was short-listed for five hospitals; she took the post of matron at Queen Elizabeth Hospital, Birmingham. She recalled her sister's preparatory words:

> You know what they say about matrons, that they are all battleaxes? Well, we have got to do something about it.

Early in her post as matron, Miss Scott determined that the role depended upon good relationships between the House Governor, Chairman, and the Medical Committee, but her primary concern was to cover the wards with sufficient staff and make herself known. She regarded the hospital as a chain; if one of the links was damaged, the whole running of the hospital could break down. Ward rounds released her from the confines of her office, but they were hard work. The hospital chain had many links, so she needed to visit the kitchen, boiler house, gardeners, engineers, laundry and linen rooms, all so that the staff could know her, and she know them. Every week she held a ward sisters' meeting, so that everyone knew what was going on.

Miss Scott points out that people today tend to forget that it could be enormous fun in a hospital, and Christmas time especially could be quite magical. One year she was lovingly caricatured at the Christmas Concert, to the delight of the audience. She saw it as a tremendous compliment. Miss Scott was not averse to joining in the fun and festivities herself, either. 'On one occasion, the sisters were preparing to do the Charleston in the Christmas show. I very stupidly said, "Oh I used to do the Charleston", so they roped me in.' On the night of the show she had to sit with the board of governors in the front row and had therefore, to work out a way of getting into her costume, so she was called to the telephone, and this was her cue to go and change. 'Of course, when it [was] time to go on the stage with all the sisters, the roof nearly went off. Do they have fun like this today? It was great fun, even though everyone worked so hard.'

For Miss Scott, the ward rounds were social, not clinical, events. It was an important part of seeing what was going on with the patients and staff, gauging the atmosphere. One important aspect of her work was training deputy and assistant matrons. Unlike her own matron, who had considered training unnecessary, Miss Scott would give anyone showing the potential ample opportunity to further their career. Miss Scott was not at all a stereotypical matron. Without a doubt her greatest asset has been her wonderful and mischievous sense of humour. 'You cannot get through life without one,' she says. Miss Scott continued to work at the Queen Elizabeth Hospital for over six years, and on two occasions was privileged to be presented to HRH the Queen Mother. The Nursing Officer of the Regional Hospital Board requested that Miss Scott apply for the matron post at Selly Oak Hospital in Birmingham. Used to a challenge, she accepted. 'It was a vertical assent.' The buildings were old and caused some serious headaches in terms of management, nevertheless she remained there for eight years until her retirement.

Miss Fraser-Gamble returned to St Mary's Hospital, London, as a ward sister and then as deputy matron. She finally accepted the prestigious post of Matron at the Hammersmith Hospital, London. She knew that fostering good relationships between herself, the Hospital Governor and Medical Superintendent was most important, especially because her appointment coincided with a period of rapid change at the hospital. Miss Fraser-Gamble made her mark on the treatment of renal patients, and was directly involved with the setting up of the first kidney transplant unit in Britain. She also held a crucial role in the development of a specialized unit for renal transplant in leukaemia patients. By now Hammersmith Hospital was considered to be a centre of excellence and innovation, and Miss Fraser-Gamble helped make this happen.

As matron, Miss Fraser-Gamble needed to keep abreast of all that was happening in the hospital. It was vital that she knew where difficulties were likely to arise, and the ward round was an effective means of ensuring this was the case. Through these rounds, she felt she had first-hand knowledge of what was going on, she could see if standards of cleanliness were being maintained, and could discover for herself how the patients were faring. Miss Fraser-Gamble's other roles were to manage the nursing budget, and to see that the wards were properly staffed. As nurse leader, she had the final say – nobody could veto her and she was answerable only to the Chairman of the Board of Governors. 'Mind you, on one occasion I went over budget by £3,000, and the Chairman of the Finance Committee was most severe with me. I had to give an undertaking that it would not happen again.'

For Miss Cooper it was a steady climb up the promotion ladder. She spent eighteen very happy months as an assistant tutor at Manchester before moving on to Bolton, where she became assistant matron. She stayed there until 1960, when she was appointed matron at Bridgewater Hospital, Eccles. Bridgewater Hospital catered for both geriatric and psychiatric patients. In total, there were four hundred beds. Miss Cooper had three assistant matrons on the geriatric side, and an assistant matron and assistant chief male nurse for the psychiatric side. Bridgewater was a lovely hospital, but there were two problems on the psychiatric unit that she had to deal with very rapidly. First, there was the issue of patients being fastened to chairs and commodes. Many nurses will have been familiar with this practice and also the restraint chairs designed to restrict patients' movements. Ending this treatment of patients proved to be difficult since it went against years of custom and practice. The second issue was about patients' clothing. At one time, patients were provided with thick, heavy, shapeless suits and dresses, and clumsy boots and shoes. It was quite a challenge to persuade the management committee of the necessity to provide individually styled (off the peg) clothing, but success in this area had a significant effect on morale. On the geriatric wards, staff also had to adopt similar courtesies instead of leaving their patients in pyjamas and ugly dressing-gowns all day.

Miss Cooper was appointed area nursing officer at Rochdale with the grand and cumbersome title of Area Nurse Local Authority Liaison, Minor Capital Planning. There were ninety-two area health authorities in the country, so she had joined 'a very select band'. She recalls the thrill of being invited to join the Matrons' Association. To her, the members were a special breed. They included Dame Muriel Powell, Dame Phyllis Friend, and matrons of the big London teaching hospitals. She felt rather small and out of place in comparison, and committed the 'sin' of attending her first national conference without a hat! Miss Cooper became Treasurer of the local matrons' association, and was awarded an MBE for her great contribution to nursing. She also helped organize four national conferences – two for the Royal College of Nursing, and two for the Association of Nurse Administrators; these were major undertakings. In 1962, she became a member of the British Institute of Management on the strength of her matron job description, and also President of the local branch of the Association of

Welfare and Hospital Administrators, because all aspects of management and administration were an everyday part of a matron's role. With her ebullient sense of humour, and a gleeful twinkle of her eye, she adds, 'By the way, I hold a unique record which will never be broken. As matron, I was trapped between two floors in a broken-down lift in the company of two Lord Mayors, their Mayoresses, and the local MP. This was on two successive Christmas Days. It played havoc with their time schedule. Now you can't beat that!'

The job Miss Mullin had been waiting for became available at Christie Hospital in 1964. Being already familiar with the hospital, and interested in the care of terminally ill patients, she was appointed Matron. In this role, she worked directly with the Medical Director and Hospital Secretary. Because of the nature of the work, and the leadership of Miss Mullin, the hospital kept up its traditional family atmosphere and its unique ability to retain its staff. Although cleanliness, hygiene, and nursing skills were highly important, other attributes were equally prized, such as compassion and empathy, dedication and understanding. The hospital thrived with an environment where morale was high and where staff were comfortable with their work. As matron, Miss Mullin always carried a bunch of keys with her which she would rattle to forewarn staff in a subtle manner that she was about. She deplored the idea of sneaking up on staff to catch them out. She respected her staff as much as they respected her.

There was a ward round every morning, where every patient was spoken to either by Miss Mullin, or one of her assistants. The ward was always informed when a round was about to commence as the nurses were often busy and it was not always appropriate to take them away from what they were doing. The rounds were important – the matron could not continually rely on others for information, and the nurses could not always remember to bring every detail to her attention. Many years later, when she was Chief Nursing Officer, Miss Mullin still went round the hospitals every month; it was her way of finding out what was going on. She was aware that at times her rounds were resented, but she needed to do them for her work.

Miss Beveridge was appointed assistant matron at Gloucester and Newcastle hospitals, and then matron of Hope Hospital, Salford. As was the case with many hospitals, Hope Hospital had difficulties in recruiting student nurses. Miss Beveridge recognized that to overcome this problem she would need more tutorial staff, so she immediately set about encouraging trained nurses to gain the necessary qualifications to become tutors and clinical teachers. In this way she carried the banner for continual, high-quality training within the nursing profession. She was rewarded with an appointment, by the General Nursing Council, to sit on the Area Nurse Training Committee, which involved visiting hospitals and reviewing nurse training throughout the region. Miss Beveridge was then appointed Chairman of the Interviewing Committee, and in this role interviewed all the candidates who wished to become tutors or clinical nurse teachers.

The Board of Governors of Charing Cross Hospital, appointed Miss Schurr as matron of Fulham Hospital in 1959. At only thirty-six years of age, Miss Schurr was one of the youngest matrons. It was to be her role to prepare the nursing service for the new Charing Cross Hospital, which was to be completed on a site in Fulham. She arrived armed with the values she had learned early on in her career. Her previous experience with Nissen hut nursing proved extremely useful because the site was nothing short of a bombsite, but Miss Schurr was not even remotely fazed by conditions there. She very quickly established professional units of a good standard in the temporary buildings. She took this opportunity to establish 'team nursing', a concept with which she had always felt comfortable. This enabled the nurses to be responsible for the total care of patients and to learn new techniques. However, she was very much aware of the delicate negotiations that would need to take place if changes were to be implemented successfully. Nursing standards were high, and the staff and people of Fulham were proud of their hospital;

Miss Schurr did not want to upset the balance.[1] The transition towards taking on the full responsibilities and activities of a teaching hospital created much additional work, but both the medical and nursing staff met these demands with enthusiasm and goodwill. Due to the nature of nurse education at the time, there was much liaison with and help from the school of nursing.

Miss Schurr had helped to create one of our country's very best hospitals, yet despite her heavy responsibilities, she still took ward rounds every morning and evening. Although not everyone could be approached, the rounds provided a valuable opportunity for her to stop and listen to a worried patient, or maybe sit for a few minutes beside someone who was very ill. Simple bedside compassion was an enduring aspect of Matron Schurr's skill. Checking on the welfare of the patients had another advantage; any requirements for extra help could be readily identified and acted upon.

In the early 1970s, more organizational and structural changes in nurse management were afoot. The Salmon Structure set out plans specifically relating to the reorganization of the nursing management structure, and our matrons were charged with implementing the required changes, even though the report was later to be linked with their own demise.

Miss Cooper was appointed Rochdale's first, and last, Director of Nursing Services. She felt that there was a great deal of misunderstanding about the Salmon report, which was to provide a new structure for nursing. It graded senior nursing staff from No. 7 Nursing Officer, to No. 10 Chief Nursing Officer. Many staff became fixated with the numbers, and Salmon was blamed for the loss of the matron role, although one small section of the report states that a suitable title for a female at Grade 9 would be 'Principal Matron'. People latched on to the new numbers without thinking them through to their logical conclusion; all they saw was that this numerical hierarchy eroded their own integrity. The report was rushed out and presented in the usual bewildering government jargon, and people simply failed to implement it properly. It was blamed for the loss of the matron title, and despite the reference regarding a Grade 9 nursing officer mentioned earlier, this could be viewed as a just criticism, because that fleeting recommendation for using the title 'Principal Matron' was buried deep within the report's pages.

As Director of Nursing Services, it was Miss Cooper's job to implement a lot of changes in a short time. Resentments ran high when people in powerful positions realized that they, too, would have to apply for their own jobs. In fact, Miss Cooper's job disappeared, as did all the other directors of nursing services; it was a time of upheaval for everyone. Accustomed to change, and with a wonderful sense of humour, she actually thought the process was a lot of fun. It was a very social affair as the application process seemed to draw the same people together time after time.

Miss Fraser-Gamble, like many senior nurses at the time, did not entirely agree with the proposals set out in the Salmon report. Accepting that it gave stronger representation for nurses, she did not agree with taking away the matron title and uniform. She felt that the strong central figure in nursing had disappeared overnight.

Miss Mullin, Miss Beveridge and Miss Schurr, equipped with their new Salmon titles of 'Chief Nursing Officer', embraced the new NHS ideology as best they could. Miss Schurr, using her teaching experience, worked hard to equip nurse managers for the advent of the Salmon recommendations prior to her own appointment. With responsibility for the nursing services of two general hospitals and five specialized hospitals, she helped pave the way for a smooth implementation.

Miss Beveridge, in a similar way to Miss Fraser-Gamble, felt unsettled by the changes imposed on her own role by the Salmon report. As Area Nursing Officer, Miss Beveridge's duties were now far more administrative, and it became more difficult for her to maintain the level of contact that she wanted with the patients and staff. This was a situation she deeply regretted, but Miss Beveridge also understood the nature of change, and embraced it. Having worked in so many hospitals, and visited others with differing standards, made her appreciate how lucky she was to have received such sound, second-to-none training. After forty years in the NHS, she looked back on the many changes that had taken place, some good, some questionable, and said, 'But with the tremendous advances taking place, one had to accept change – it was time to look forward.'

As Chief Nursing Officer to the North Sheffield University Hospital Management Committee, Miss Mullin's responsibilities spanned a large group of hospitals across the city. The Northern General and Firvale hospitals were older model hospitals. Firvale had originally been a workhouse infirmary, and was separated from the General Hospital by a large brick wall. Miss Mullin was charged not only with the responsibility for introducing the new Salmon management structure, but also with removing the 'wall' culture that so threatened the new NHS team ethos. It proved to be a far harder task than anticipated, and she encountered consider-able resistance. Trade unions had started to assert their influ-ence, and senior posts were becoming less clinical and more administrative. Miss Mullin decided that the time had come to leave the politics of nursing behind; she, like the other matrons in this chapter, felt unable to see through to fruition another raft of changes. It seemed the right time for someone else to take the helm. In purely practical terms, the person implementing change in a long-term strategy should be the one charged with planning it.

All of our esteemed contributors retired between the ages of fifty-five and sixty years. They had devoted the best part of their working lives to nursing, and their reminiscences still resonate with the vibrancy of this competent and caring profession. These women are wise; they are the people we need to listen to and learn from before they, too, slip into the mists of history. A little older now, these women still maintain an active involvement in community life, and a critical inter-est in the current hospital and nursing services. They have watched the National Health Service heave, change and falter.

Accepting the necessity of change, they still question the wisdom of dropping matrons from nursing.

Note

1. Schurr, Margaret M.C. (ed.) *The Nurses at Fulham* (The Fulham Nurses' League, London, 1996)

XV
Last of the Dinosaurs

Miss Hirons was one of the very last matrons to stay in her uniform and proudly keep her title. Against a tide of organizational change and new managerial titles, she remained a clearly identified nurse leader, in her uniform and with the patient at the centre of her care orchestration.

Miss Ann Hirons was born in 1933 at Kingswinford, only eight miles from where she lives now – she is undoubtedly a 'Black Country lass, and proud of it!' She took three A levels in history, English and geography at Stourbridge High School; this was some achievement as they were the first A levels ever to be taken. Because Ann was leaving school after the war, her head teacher still had doubts about nursing as a career, and would have preferred for her to have gone on to university. Ann would have loved to do a history degree before commencing nursing, simply for pleasure, but this was not possible then, besides which, family finances did not allow it. Her family life had been devastated when her father was killed in an accident in 1944; Ann Hirons was just eleven years old. As a result of the death, Ann and her brother Dick, who later trained to be an accountant, became very close. Miss Hirons' own mother had longed to be a nurse, but as she had a mother who did not enjoy the best of health, she had remained at home to nurse her. Obviously she was delighted when her only daughter entered nursing.

In 1951, when Miss Hirons started nurse training at Wolverhampton Royal Hospital, sugar and sweets were still subject to rationing, the last of the post-war shortages. The nurses' home was also a bit spartan, reflecting the legacy of the recent past, but Ann loved the camaraderie. As a group, the nurses would get all their frustrations off their chests over steaming mugs of coffee or tea. 'We still had to be in by ten, but it was such fun. You hated sleeping on the lower floor because of the pebbles that used to be thrown at the window by nurses coming back late. After lights out we would sit on the bed with a drink, in the dark so night sister did not see, and we would have a good gossip.'

At her training hospital, the student nurses were often thrown in at the deep end. At one point, Miss Hirons was put in charge of the accident and emergency department of the hospital. She had to stitch everything except faces, take blood samples, set fractures (not unusual in provincial hospitals), and she was only a second year nurse! It surprised her, therefore, when she commenced her midwifery training at the Simpson Memorial Pavilion in Edinburgh, and found herself to be far ahead of the other nurses from the major teaching hospitals in terms of practical experience. This earned her a great deal of respect from most of the medical staff. When she was a ward sister, however, and when the consultant was on his way, she admits to having said, 'Look out, God is coming', but at the bed the consultant would always say, 'What do you think, Sister?' and her advice was almost always taken.

If Miss Hirons has a worry, it is that nurses now do not seem to have this same practical training. Nursing, she feels, does have to move on, and a lot of the changes made do make sense, but she wonders if there should not be more consideration given to basic care, including hygiene. She once called to a doctor, 'Sir, you have not washed your hands.' She directed him to the sink, and made sure he washed them. 'What ward sister would do that now?' she asked. As the ward sister, she knew everything about each patient.

Miss Hirons's road to promotion continued; she spent a period as a night superintendent, then as an assistant matron, and then a year at the Staff College for Matrons in London. This was followed by two years at the Royal Hospital in Sheffield, where she was deputy matron. After this, she returned to the Midlands, as matron of Kidderminster General Hospital. She worked at the hospital for two years, opening various phases of the hospital's development, and overseeing the small hospital when it became a modern geriatric unit. She gained invaluable experience. Because of the Salmon changes, the job title changed to Principal Nursing Officer. She was responsible for Kidderminster, Bromsgrove and Droitwich, and a number of small cottage hospitals. It was another unsettling time, not because of a lack of support, but because it was a job without identity; Miss Hirons fitted in nowhere, driving round visiting all those hospitals. She was very hesitant about another move. Miss Hirons did not want to move her mother, who was by now quite ill, but her mother said in a typical manner, 'My life is nearly over, yours lies before you. As long as I am with you, that's all that matters.' Ann's mother had been a constant support to her throughout her career. On one occasion when she was still a student nurse, Ann returned from leave to find she had been allocated back to theatre. Theatre was not an experience she had enjoyed. She went back upstairs to her mother and said, 'I can't bear it, I have to go back to theatre and I hate it.' Her mother replied, 'Get on with it, don't be silly. You have just got to get on with it' – and that was that!

Miss Hirons has known many matrons during her training, ranging from the very gentle to the harsh ones. She learned a great deal from them all, incorporating these lessons into her own work as matron. A lot can be told about the nature of Miss Hirons because once she was almost destroyed by one matron, but managed to overcome it and still learnt lessons from it. 'I sort of mix and matched, taking the good bits and the bad bits.' Her greatest influence was Muriel Lee, a ward sister at the David Lewis Northern Hospital, Liverpool. She worked with 'Tubby' Lee (as she was known), who was a most outstanding ward sister. A very strict disciplinarian, Tubby was a wonderful influence on Ann's career, and virtually her professional mentor, a term Tubby Lee finds strange. Tubby Lee taught the importance of cleanliness, 'My word, you would not have cross-infection on Tubby's ward, nor bedsores may I add!' Weekends on the ward were spent cleaning everything; every trolley, every tray would be cleaned, and the nurses were proud of it. Because they didn't have such things as CSSD (Central Sterile Supply Department), cleanliness was essential, everything had to be boiled. The ward maids were directly under the ward sister's direction, so she would check that the ward sluice and kitchen were neat, tidy and clean. Today, a catheter, for example, is taken from a plastic wrapper and thrown away after it has been used, but back then the nurses had to boil the rubber tubing. 'A far cry from washing out an old cordial bottle, putting the tube in, and tying it to the bed. But patient care was always uppermost.'

Miss Hirons returned to the Wolverhampton Royal Hospital and quickly gained a promotion from staff nurse to ward sister. These were probably the five happiest years of her nursing career. The post was offered to her by matron, and she did not have to apply. 'The matron could do that then. I never could, there was too much legislation by the time I became matron.' She did have to face considerable disappointment, however, when she was instructed to introduce the first intensive care unit to the hospital, because it was not received too readily. This made for a very hard few months. Miss Hirons also had two difficult years as assistant matron, but she battled through. From this she vowed she would learn as many lessons as possible, and she did, 'My time as an assistant matron was the most difficult; I belonged to nothing, I had control over nothing, and I felt completely lost.'

Miss Hirons was appointed Principal Nursing Officer (Matron) of the Birmingham General Hospital in April 1973. With her usual sense of fun she described the interview: 'It was the last time I ever wore a hat for an interview. Of course, being a "lady", I always wore one when I attended the matron's association. As a preliminary to the interview, one had to perform the usual acrobatics by demonstrating the art of balancing the buffet lunch in one hand, a glass of sherry in the other, and eating at the same time.' The first thing she did when she commenced her post was to disconnect the bell between her office and the outer office. This was the bell that matron used when summoning a nurse. The fearsome sound of it still resonated in her own ears, so she knew how hated it was. She also reversed the desk, never again sitting behind it to interview staff. Gone was the row of filing cabinets; in its place were comfortable chairs, potted plants and impressionist paintings. She served endless coffee, and had a bottle of sherry for special occasions, which 'got many a thing through the hospital committee'.

It was at once clear to Miss Hirons that her immediate senior did not want her to wear a matron's uniform, so she forwent her cap to begin with, and just wore a plain navy dress. She knew she had to tread carefully, but after twelve months she put her cap back on. She did not wear the uniform every day, but always when she was in the hospital; otherwise she wore a tailored suit. 'I soon sized things up and realized that my role as matron was important to the General. I had about fifty to sixty per cent of sisters that I called my 'navy matriarchs'. These sisters were still in navy, the material being paid for by one of the old consultants.'

Miss Hirons would soon feel fortunate that she had been on a management course at Henley Administrative Staff College, which was compared favourably with the Harvard Business School. She was one of only three women on the course, but there were sixty-eight men. Her section still meets after twenty-five years. This learning helped her to assess, shape, and define the roles of nursing and administration; it also showed her more clearly the role played by trade unions in the health service. One leading militant figure had infiltrated the health service unions, and by 1973 the unions were very active. Miss Hirons found herself in the basement doing business in smoke-filled rooms. The nurses at one point were reduced to using paper bed-sheets, and because Miss Hirons had seen a patient die of terrible jaundice in these papers sheets, she vowed it was to be the last time. 'I said to the branch secretary, for whom I had great respect, "Never let me see that happen again", and, give him credit, it never did.' The course at Henley College was also supposed to be part of her grooming for the next Chief Nurse position in Birmingham, but it had the opposite effect on her. 'That course taught me that this post was not for me.'

Retaining her uniform and title until she retired, Miss Hirons firmly believed that the matron uniform, including its 'frilly hat', was a necessary mark of identification in the ever-changing hospital world. Seeing her role as the figurehead, she felt the uniform made her immediately identifiable to patients and visitors to the hospital. She would wear the tailored suit to meetings, both in and outside the hospital. Her traditional matron's uniform was the symbol of her total dedication to nursing, and her tailored suit affirmed modernization and administrative progress.

When she started the post at the General Hospital, she found that the No. 7 Nursing Officer grade was often looked down upon as 'dirty'. Some of the people in that post were clinically inadequate, but by the time Miss Hirons left, she felt that the grade was respected. By that time, people who could do the job were placed in the posts. 'The consultants had to learn to go to the nursing officers, not me, and of course it took several years to introduce my own clinically competent nursing officers, but I expected to act down as much as they acted up.'

Miss Hirons is rightly proud that she was matron of a hospital that spanned two centuries. Looking back at the great people who had built the hospital and the remarkable staff who had run it, she feels privileged to have been a matron. 'They left a tradition that I could build on.' In 1979 it was the bicentenary of the Birmingham General Hospital, and there was a memorial service in the cathedral, followed by a perfor-mance of Mendelssohn's *Elijah* in the Town Hall. Other fundraising events included the bicentenary fair, run by the nursing staff. The funds raised helped to provide for opportu-nities in medical research, and Miss Hirons saw that some of the funds went to scholarships for nurses.

Regular daily contact with the staff and patients was essential; it was the purpose of 'doing the rounds'. These rounds were not like the ones she remembers, where the nurses were petrified, but a means of exchanging views on patient care. The most important person to her was the patient. 'When I did my round, I usually went on my own. I just wandered around and chatted, then I would have a cup of tea with the ward sister.' This courtesy and informality extended to other departments, where she would sit with staff, chat over a coffee, thank them if they had made an extra effort with something, or discuss issues they felt were important; this was a style that required trust. Miss Hirons's door was always open, and staff could meet with her at any time. She much preferred dealing with problems face to face rather than on the telephone. 'I would use up shoe leather by getting out into the corridors and wards, or having people come to me. Many a problem has been solved in the corridor.' While standards of care and cleanliness were still of the utmost importance, it was also important to understand the problems that staff faced, 'To ensure they were able to uphold the standards set; I could only find this out by first-hand experience.'

August each year was acting down time for Miss Hirons. She knew things were fairly quiet, so she would don the uniform of an enrolled nurse, and for three or four days be allocated as a nurse to a team. In this role she did drug rounds, and it was through doing this that she realized that surgical drug rounds were just as busy as medical rounds. When acting down she still had the chance to show old skills. One of the patients on a ward had bone cancer and was dying; he longed to have his hair washed. The nurses were unsure about how to deal with this. As a student, she had taken the back off the bed many a time for this procedure, and had also had her own hair washed this way in the practical room. 'So I said, "Right, take the back of the bed off", and we washed his hair.' The students could not believe their matron was doing that. Miss Hirons feels she could not be a 'high-tech nurse' now, but equally believes she could make a patient more comfortable in bed, make sure their meals were given, and keep their mouths clean.

The biggest incident in Miss Hirons's life occurred on the night of 21 November 1974. All the events of her nursing career came together on that night. The event was the Birmingham pub bombing, and it caused the largest number of casualties on the mainland so far since the Northern Ireland troubles began.

Miss Hirons had been at the General Hospital, attending a party for voluntary workers. The party was just finishing when they heard a big thud, but they did not consider it might be anything sinister. Miss Hirons sent Helen Tees, who was to be her deputy, to go and find out what was happening. It was known that an IRA terrorist had blown himself up in an explosion in Coventry the previous week, so they had been alerted to the possibilities of trouble, and services were already in place to deal with any emergencies, but on that night the first people to arrive on the scene were taxi drivers. They started to bring in the injured before any alerts had been given. 'All your nursing life you are taught how to deal with major catastrophes. Fortunately, the night staff were just coming on duty so we had a reasonable complement of nurses, but there were no consultants. So I grabbed a white coat and some "theatre pumps", as I still had my party dress on.'

With an event such as this, one has to think on the spot and get organized. Miss Hirons decided that the 'five-day patients' ward could be used to make bed space for the injured, and she put Helen Tees in charge of that. Then she went round the hospital alerting the areas that she knew would be needed: X-ray, intensive care, and the operating theatres. All the day staff stayed on duty, and she moved them to key areas. Miss Hirons put another nursing officer in charge of the dining room, in readiness for relatives. Consultants did not start to arrive until much later, due to the centre of Birmingham being cordoned off, but they were happy with the arrangements. When the senior physician asked Miss Hirons how he could help, she told him to open the pharmacy. Miss Hirons stayed until half past five in the morning, going round each area, helping with any crisis as it arose, making sure that the staff were coping, and moving them around to other areas accordingly. Not realizing just how tired she was becoming, Ann did not stop until one of the consultants intervened. It was at about one in the morning when she had just gone to theatre to see if everyone was managing. One of the consultants came along, pushed her into a chair, and asked one of the nurses to make a sweet cup of tea for matron. 'I said, "Jimmy, I do not take sugar", but he made me drink this huge mug of hot, sweet tea. I think he realized that I had taken the brunt of it and that I needed to stop for a few minutes. Afterwards, he wrote me two of the most moving letters I ever had.'

As staff arrived, Miss Hirons directed them to areas of most need. It was all systems go. Miss Hirons saw sights that night the likes of which she hopes never to see again. People were brought in with their limbs blown off. It was the worst atrocity to happen on the mainland. Twenty-one people died, and between the general and the accident hospitals, over a hundred casualties were taken in. To add to the atrocity, there had been napalm in the bombs, aimed at causing maximum burns. Miss Hirons took two parents into the five-day ward where their son had just come from theatre. They could barely see his eyes because he was swathed in bandages. She took the parents to the bed, and as soon as the mother saw him she became hysterical, saying 'That is not my son!' Miss Hirons knew the mother's need at that moment was greater than the boy's, so she gently touched him and said, 'Can you tell me your name?' He repeated his name, and then the mother realized he was her son. Miss Hirons found that moment deeply moving, and the meaning of the dreadful events of that night came home to her.

The response from the nurses in Birmingham had been tremendous. The emergency had galvanized the whole hospital, and in the end Miss Hirons was overwhelmed by the level of support she received. She pointed out: 'The spirit in the General was just fantastic; I can't praise them enough, they were totally professional.' Although she had been in the post for only twelve months, she felt the experience cemented her in the heart of the hospital. Miss Hirons lived at the hospital for those five days. When she got home, the shock of those few days hit her. She talked to her brother, who was wonderful. She also realized just how much she missed talking to her mother, who had died only six months previously.

Miss Hirons was asked many times how she and her nurses coped without the benefits of counselling. She says, 'In 1974 there was no such thing as counselling for nurses; we did not have counsellors. So, having been on our feet for twenty-four hours, we went to the nurses' home, kicked our shoes off, made a drink, and talked. We supported each other – the spirit of comradeship was tremendous. I do not know of any staff casualties because of the traumas. It brought out the best in people.' She feels her experience as a second-year nurse on casualty, having the accidents and the drunks to deal with, stood her in good stead.

The Duke of Edinburgh, Prince Philip, arrived that Monday to visit the injured and the hospital staff. He made it clear that it was to be an informal occasion, and he wanted no fuss. When Miss Hirons and the Duke were walking along the corridor, along came 'little Frank', the rubbish disposal man, who was so important within the hospital. As they walked past, Frank said, 'Morning, Matron. Morning, Sir.' – he had no idea who 'Sir' was! At the end of his visit they found they had another ten minutes to spare. Prince Philip asked if there were any other staff that she would like him to meet, so she pointed out Mrs Evans. Mrs Evans was the nursing officer who had been working so hard behind the scenes with the relatives. The Queen visited the following March, which was again a very proud moment for the hospital. This was a more formal occasion.

A letter of appreciation from the medical staff was written to Miss Hirons on 23 November 1974. It read:

Dear Miss Hirons,
    The medical staff were full of admiration for the way you handled everything in the hospital after the three bombs exploded.
    Most of us arrived when all was organized and patients were already being treated. Ward five was a model of foresight.

Everywhere were sisters, nurses and many other people, and everywhere the Matron seemed to be appearing from nowhere.

I know all this would have been impossible without the loyal support of your staff, but such support grew rapidly after your appointment.

This letter is written to convey to you, and to all your Sisters and Nurses, the very sincere appreciation and thanks of the medical staff.

Yours sincerely,

M.B.

Back to more routine activities at the hospital, Miss Hirons now had the Matrons' Ball to organize. This was originally a Christmas Ball, then it became an annual Midsummer Ball attended by any staff. Dinner jackets were deliberately not stipulated so that the Ball could be open to anyone. Miss Hirons always stood on the stairs to greet the guests. As she had no partner, Mr John Baron, a member of the Area Health Authority, regularly escorted her. These occasions were important events, providing an opportunity for staff to socialize and enjoy themselves, with matron prepared to 'jig with the best of them'.

With the help of the Chairman of the League of Friends, the link between the City of Birmingham Orchestra and the General Hospital was revived, satisfying the great love of Ann Hirons's life: music. Her time at the General Hospital coincided with the 'young' Simon Rattle (now Sir Simon) being appointed the conductor; Miss Hirons has had the great joy of watching him establish the City of Birmingham Symphony Orchestra on the world stage.

The Sisters' Dinner followed the Christmas festivities and was held in the boardroom. The main guest was the Chairman of the Medical Staff Committee. Miss Hirons has kept all the speeches she made. This dinner involved writing the most difficult speech of the year; she was always expected to be funny. The house men waited on them, and at times it was difficult to keep order. With the drink flowing, bread rolls did occasionally fly across the room when matron was not look-ing! She was always anxious that no missile from the other tables should hit the consultants next to her. 'I always had to take the mickey out of the medical staff committee chairman, so I used to pick on [his] idiosyncrasies. Not too difficult!'

It must be noted that there have never been any awards given to any of the personnel involved in helping the injured of the Birmingham bombing. In 1987, however, the Regional Nursing Officer nominated Miss Hirons for the MBE, as thanks for her services to nursing. After this, many people felt that justice had been done. Following the award ceremony at the palace, Miss Hirons's brother and his wife, along with two friends, took her to the Ritz. The Ritz staff had already been informed of the occasion, and they asked Miss Hirons what she would like them to play. She requested 'I Could Have Danced All Night' from *My Fair Lady*. To the accompani-ment of the violin, Miss Hirons sang:

> I could have danced all night,
> I could have danced all night,
> And still come back for more . . .
> I only know when she
> Put the gong on me,
> I could have danced, danced, danced
> All night.

As part of the Christmas show, the nurses performed a sketch about Miss Hirons's visit to the palace. One of the staff had taken notes at the informal talk Miss Hirons had given, where she described the events at the palace. 'It was unbelievable to me; great fun.' It was intended as fun, but it also gave an opportunity for Miss Hirons to thank her nursing staff for all their support. It saddens Miss Hirons that much of the joy she experienced seems to have gone out of the modern health service.

Miss Hirons recognizes that Birmingham General Hospital was part of a great tradition, and is proud of the torch of caring that they were fortunate enough to inherit. She can also see the need for change. Prior to 1986, there had been three equals running the hospital: the Adminstrator, the Chairman of the Staff Committee, and the Senior Nurse, or Matron. After the report on general management, many ex-servicemen were introduced as general managers. Brigadier Brian Thomas CBE, formerly Provost Marshal of the Military Police, was appointed to the general hospital. As he had no background in the health service at all, but was a very able manager, he was pleased to retain Miss Hirons in the matron role, and was very proud to introduce her as 'his' matron. Miss Hirons was appointed his deputy, and in this role she was also responsible for the doctors' mess. 'Now that was interesting!' she says with a smile. She continued her role until her retirement in 1989. On her retirement day, she was given a memorable send-off, and afterwards was presented with a video of the occasion. The great regard the staff held Miss Hirons in is clearly apparent from this video, and the speeches described a remarkable career and a wonderful person.

The day after she retired in 1989, Miss Hirons was admitted to the Rheumatology Unit of Droitwich Hospital. She stayed for nine weeks. One day she was a matron, the next she was a patient! She had learned to 'put on a good face' whilst matron, but now had to accept that she would need treatment. It is her nature to push herself; even now she visits and helps others in spite of her arthritic problems. 'I can't let my old people down.' After thirty-eight and a half years in nursing, Miss Hirons could say that the three things that stood her in good stead throughout her career were her good sense of humour, her family, and her Christian faith. Through her faith, she saw all of her work as a vocation. 'In my day the word "vocation" did not have the lamentable connotations it seems to have today.'

Although she was an undoubted success in the career she chose, Miss Hirons did not fulfil all of her ambitions in life. 'I never wanted to be a career girl. Being very maternal, I really wanted to be a wife and a mother, but I never let myself become embittered because of that. I am terribly grateful that I had such a wonderful career, a career where I could be so fulfilled.' The history of the hospital was important to her, and she was able not only to preserve its traditions, but also to be the matron who introduced modern management. The two greatest highs of her career were the five years during which she was ward sister at Wolverhampton, and the time she was matron of the Birmingham General Hospital. 'I was made for the General, and the General was made for me. It gave me what I was looking for, and I was able to give back what the General Hospital was looking for. In the end I felt I had my family there; they were my family.'

After the retirement of Miss Hirons, the era of traditional nurse leadership was over. The National Health Service is now a modern and complex organization, with a hard-to-define and self-perpetuating management structure. There is no longer a place for the unique nurse leader, the Matron. Living on only in the minds of those who search through archives in search of information about them, matron has become the hospital dinosaur. This is a crying shame; over many decades, matrons showed great adaptability, and enthusiasm for change. Matron had been flexible to meet new demands and challenges, but without compromising standards in nursing. Matrons were the much-respected and feared giants of hospitals, the stalwart leaders of nursing. Like many other things in our careless modern world, matrons were unable to survive the climate of change, a change to a new organizational and management structure of nursing. This happened despite matrons having been so instrumental in moulding British nursing into a profession admired and copied throughout the world.

XVI

The Values We Took with Us

It would be wrong to judge the nursing standards of the past by the standards of the twenty-first century, however the underlying principles and values of nursing have changed little since Florence Nightingale's time. From the people interviewed in this book, it would appear that the fundamentals of traditional nursing were discipline, orderliness, cleanliness, and a desire to help people and relieve suffering.

Discipline was inherent in both the religious and military roots of nursing. These roots formed the basis of the nursing hierarchy, and some of the titles. The authority of matron, and the centralization of nursing to one person, formed the foundation of modern nursing. Orderliness was an essential prerequisite for the day-to-day running of a hospital; neatness and tidiness were necessary for the wards and equipment; spotless uniforms reflected the hygiene and propriety of the nurses. Cleanliness was the barrier to infection; the cleaning of wards, the changing of aprons, the washing of hands, and the proper use of aseptic techniques were central to fighting against infections. Hygiene was paramount and understood by all the staff of the hospital.

Mike Owen, a community mental health nurse, and Steve Moss, Director of Nursing and Patient Services, Queen's Medical Centre, Nottingham, were reminiscing about their nursing experiences. Inevitably the conversation focused on the comparisons between old and new hospital customs and organization. Steve Moss pointed out, 'I think we probably gained most from the values our matrons left with us, but of course it was a different culture!' Both men are nurses at heart, and neither will relinquish his nursing background. Although he misses hands-on clinical nursing, Steve Moss finds that he can still influence the quality of care that patients receive by building into the job descriptions of all nurses in management a half-day per week for them to work in the patient areas. Mike Owens finds his work in the community with children influenced by the values he learned through nurse training.

Lynette King summed up the rule of matron:

> Under Matron's ever-watchful eye, the hospital ran like clock-work; from cleaners, to kitchen staff, to surgeons, all respected her and were proud to be part of her establishment. Besides respect she was admired, and we all felt we had to do our very best for her. She did not suffer fools gladly. We knew exactly where we stood, and she certainly kept us on our toes. She was a formidable figure, yes; someone of whom you were health-ily fearful. Down-to-earth, honest, sincere, and trustworthy, she gave her nurses self-confidence, had a quick wit, and eyes in the back of her head. She had all the right qualities in the right quantities, leaving any nurse with a set of values that she can cherish to this day.

A cynic might suggest that the values matron cherished are somehow redundant in a modern society, let alone in a modern hospital system. Matron's values were based on respect, courtesy, loyalty, devotion and faith. Matrons from the Nightingale School onwards wanted the best for nursing, striving for the highest standards at their hospitals, and demanding commendable behaviour from their nurses. Matron inspired respect, but only through merit. Not all matrons were respected, and these matrons did not get the best out of their staff.

Before every Association of Hospital Matrons' meeting, the following prayer would be said:

> O God, who dost teach the world that those who lead must serve, bless the work of hospital matrons that they may ever combine gentleness with firmness, and humility with authority. Grant them wisdom and patience amid all the pressing problems of their task. Vouchsafe to them the constant sense of Thy Presence, that they may go about their work with cheerfulness and courtesy, endowed with inward peace and outward calmness. All this we ask through Jesus Christ our living, loving Lord, whose service is perfect freedom.

What was the culture that is now missed by so many nurses? It was a different culture of leadership. Nurse leadership was gained through experience and credibility. All matrons would start at the bottom, and rise through the nursing ranks, getting to know the system along the way, becoming a ward manager first and then a matron. In a partnership with the hospital secretary and medical officer, a simpler decision-making process was possible. It was a different culture of care; a patient's stay in hospital was much longer; tender loving care of the patient was central. If a patient needed assistance, any nurse would be willing, and available, to provide that help. It was also a different culture of cleaning: wards were spotless. If something was dropped on the floor, someone would pick it up; if something was dirty, it would be washed. An argument over the demarcation of duties would not have happened, and certainly would not have been tolerated by matron. It was a different culture of pride: pride in one's work, and pride in one's appearance as a nurse. Attachment to one's hospital and colleagues was forged in the training system, and in the nurses' home. Nurses served an apprenticeship in their training – they learned the job in the areas in which they worked, doing all the activities associated with the skills they needed.

The culture of support was different: nurses had their own networking systems. Hospital corridors and dining rooms were important; in them the nurses exchanged information and gained informal support. Ward teams stayed together longer, and the students learned the value of belonging. The nurses' home also had its special support role when the nurses were off duty. Fun was associated with hospital life; it permeated the atmosphere from the bottom to the top, and back again. It was fundamental to disciplined life, and inherent in the camaraderie of staff, in the relationships with patients, and was sometimes used as a defence mechanism against the suffering that nurses encountered daily. Fun was manifest in organized activities, harmless pranks ('apple pie beds!'), and in day-to-day repartee.

A culture of dedication and allegiance is more difficult to attain in a world where short-term contracts mean increasing insecurity and more movement in the workplace, especially now that nurses are educated at universities. Roy Stallard, contemplating the closure of the Wolverhampton Royal Hospital Nurses' League, identifies the problem: 'The nurse training schools we knew are long gone, having been replaced by university establishments with the more practical aspects of tuition centred on one or more hospitals or nursing homes. These features in themselves have removed the loyalty and ethos that we all enjoyed at our individual hospitals, and nurses of today no longer share this camaraderie, with organizations such as ours offering little attraction. One thing we will not lose is the sense of caring and discipline inbred into us in yesteryear, or the long warm friendships we have enjoyed.'

The anticipated loss of a nurses' league can be great, as these responses to a letter regarding the closure of Wolverhampton Royal Hospital Nurses' League show:

> How upsetting it was to read the letter, but [I] understand completely the difficulties of keeping the league going in this ever-changing world of ours . . . I say this with a sad heart, but the situation has to be faced sooner or later.
> *Sheila Waterhouse*

> It was with great sadness that I read the letter that the league will be closing on its 50th anniversary. Somehow one expects

these things will go on forever, but if closure is the only option, then this would be the ideal time. But let's enjoy what we have for the few remaining reunions ahead.

Audrey Pead (the first Nursing Officer at Wolverhampton)

This attachment to, and affection for, one's own hospital formed the basis for pride in one's work and loyalty to colleagues, and, as reflected in the above letters, it lasted long after the closure of hospitals. All reunions are times to reminisce, and hospital reunions are no different, but they do have their own special qualities. Those attending such reunions have shared a unique range of human experiences, from 'living in' to bedside care, and all the staff, of course, have stories to tell about matron!

Many hospitals may not only lose their leagues, but also their idiosyncratic languages. The 'old' Fulham Hospital language required a Fulham nurse, with the aid of historical notes, to translate it! Maria Brennan (née O'Shaughnessy) trained at Fulham Hospital, retired as a senior nurse manager, and is currently secretary of the Nurses' League. She helped explain the following terminology: 'We had "Sibs", nurses trained at the hospital, "ceorls" were the other nurses; the "Head Thane" was matron; "moot" was an assembly or meeting; and a "bond" was formed in 1918 to maintain a link for nurses.' Records state that the purpose of the 'bond' was to maintain a link in the training school for the past and present nurses, so that all may keep in contact with the hospital and its matron, seeking advice as they progress in the nursing world, also keeping in touch with their colleagues. Maintaining such strong links and attachments is difficult in an evolving nursing profession, but they unite us with nursing's historical roots.

At ninety-one years of age, Mrs Soper can still look back on and value her nursing experiences.

On reflection, the disciplined life we led must all seem rather harsh now, and sometimes extreme. It did not do us any harm and, in fact, probably prepared and strengthened us for both a

World War and our future careers. This is not being nostalgic. As a ninety-one-year-old, and very much wiser, I can appreciate the responsibility that matron had on her shoulders. Matron not only had a large hospital to run, but was also *in loco parentis* to [us] young nurses resident in the hospital. The disciplined regime ensured safety, efficiency, and high standards at all levels. [Matrons] had an enormously daunting job, but they were women of strength and character. In my day, matron was head of nursing, and had the authority. Prestigious and imposing, she led from the front. Nurses knew where they were, and who their leader was, and liked it. Will we ever see the likes of them again?

POSTSCRIPT
Modern Matron

The 'NHS Plan – Modern Matrons' initiative was issued on 4 April 2001. The paper sets out the structure, job descriptions, competencies, and strategies required to strengthen the role of all ward sisters and charge nurses, and introduces a new role for matron. The NHS paper makes it clear that 'the demand for a matron be met'.

The main aim of the paper is the introduction of a modern matron into the clinical areas. This matron will have responsibility for a number of wards, particularly as regards areas such as hygiene and the quality of hospital food. It is the matron's job to see that support service is designed and delivered to achieve the highest standards of care, and to provide a visible, accessible, and authoritative presence on the wards.

The key attributes of matron candidates will be professional credibility achieved through experience. They will also need to be respected individuals who take pride in the National Health Service, and have experience as clinical managers.

Bibliography

Able-Smith, B., *A History of the Nursing Profession* (Heinemann Educational Books, Ltd., London, 1960)

Baly, M.E., *Florence Nightingale and the Nursing Legacy* (Croom Helm, London, 1986)

Bowman, G., *The Lamp and the Book* (The Queen Ann Press, London, 1967)

Cadbury, M.C. *The Story of a Nightingale Nurse* (Headley Brothers, London, 1939)

Charles, L. and Duffin, L., *Women and Work in Pre-Industrialised England* (Croom Helm, London, 1985)

Connor, B., *A Pauper Palace: A History of Fishpool Institution* (N. Richardson, Bolton, 1989)

Cook, E.T., *The Life of Florence Nightingale*, 2 volumes, (Macmillan, London, 1913)

Davies, C., *Rewriting Nursing History* (Croom Helm, London, 1980)

Delgado, A., *As They Saw Her: Florence Nightingale* (Harrap & Co. Ltd., London, 1970)

Greene, J., *Dominic Remembers, Life in County Clare 1916 to 1935* (K. Greene, Newcastle upon Tyne, 1994)

Hamilton, N., *Monty: Master of the Battlefield 1942–1944* (Hamish Hamilton Ltd., London, 1983)

Hughes, M.J., *Women Healers in Medieval Life and Literature* (Morningside Heights, New York, 1943)

Hurd-Mead, K.C., *A History of Women in Medicine from the Earliest Times to the Beginning of the Nineteenth Century* (Haddam Press, Haddam, Connecticut, 1938)

Jamieson, E.M., Sewall, M.F., and Gjertson, L.S., *Trends in Nursing History* (Saunders & Co., London, 1959)

Jennings, W.I. *The Poor Law Code* (Charles Knight & Co. Ltd., London, circa 1930)

Kopperman, P.E., 'Medical Services in the British Army, 1742–1783' in *Journal of the History of Medicine & Allied Science Vol. XXXIV* (OUP, 1979)

MacDonnell, F., *Miss Nightingale's Young Ladies* (Angus and Robertson Ltd., London, 1970)

MacManus, E., *Matron of Guy's* (Andrew Melrose, London, 1956)

Monter, W.E., 'The Pedestal and the Stake: Courtly Love and Witchcraft' in Biedenthal, R. and Koonz, C. (eds) *Becoming Visible* (Houghton Mifflin, Boston, 1977)

Pavey, A.E., *The Story of the Growth of Nursing: as an Art, a Vocation, and a Profession* (Faber and Faber Ltd., London, 1937)

Rendall, J., *Women in Industrialising Society 1750–1880* (Blackwell, Oxford, 1990)

Richardson, R.G., *Nurse Sarah Anne* (John Murray Ltd., London, 1977)

Schurr, Margaret M.C. (ed.) *The Nurses at Fulham* (The Fulham Nurses' League, London, 1996)

Seymer, L.R., *A General History of Nursing* (Faber and Faber Ltd., London, 1932)

Smith, F.B., *Florence Nightingale, Reputation and Power* (Croom Helm Ltd., Kent, 1982)

Summers, A., *Angels and Citizens* (Routledge & Keegan Paul Ltd., London, 1989)

Vicinus, M. and Nergaard, B. (eds), *Ever Yours, Florence Nightingale* (Virago Press, London, 1989)

Woodham-Smith, C., *Florence Nightingale* (Constable and Co., London, 1950)

Yeo, G., *Nursing at Bart's* (Alan Sutton Ltd., Stroud, 1995)

Index

Index

Index